New Edition! Enlarged and Revised!

BRAGG SYSTEM OF SUPER-BRAIN BREATHING

for Health and Energy

By
PAUL C. BRAGG, N.D., Ph.D.
LIFE EXTENSION SPECIALIST

and
PATRICIA BRAGG, Ph.D.
Health and Beauty Consultant

"The Lord God formed man of the dust of the ground, and breathed into his nostrils THE BREATH OF LIFE; and man became a living soul."
—*Genesis 2:7*

This Book Can Mean
The Very Breath of Life to You!

Published by
HEALTH SCIENCE
Box 7, Santa Barbara, California 93102 U.S.A.

BRAGG SYSTEM OF SUPER-BRAIN BREATHING
for Health and Energy

By

By Paul C. Bragg, N.D., Ph.D.
Life Extension Specialist
and
Patricia Bragg, Ph.D.
Health and Beauty Consultant

Copyright © Health Science
Eighteenth Printing MCMLXXX

All rights, including the Right of translation into other languages, are reserved by the Publisher. No part of this book may be reproduced in any form, by mimeograph or any other means, without permission in writing from the Publisher.

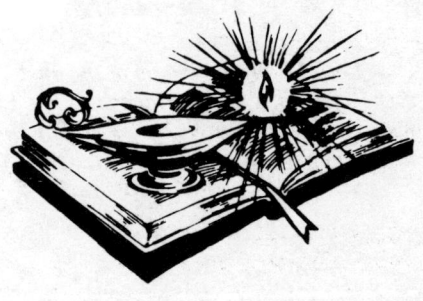

Published in the United States by

HEALTH SCIENCE Box 7, Santa Barbara, California 93102 U.S.A.

Library of Congress Catalog Card Number: 74-32637
ISBN: 0-87790-014-0
Printed in the United States of America

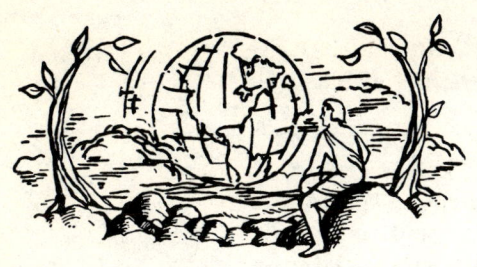

CONTENTS

CHAPTERS

1. **DO YOU KNOW HOW TO BREATHE?** 1
   Living at a High Rate of Vibration . . . Learn How to Increase Your Energy by Deep Breathing . . . Living at a Medium Rate of Vibration . . . Value of the "Second Wind" . . . Misery at a Low Rate of Vibration

2. **OXYGEN STARVATION** 5
   Oxygen Powers the Human Machine . . . Oxygen Carried by the Bloodstream . . . Purification of the Blood . . . Shallow Breathers Poison Themselves

3. **THE WAY YOU BREATHE IS THE WAY YOU LIVE** 10
   Your Marvelous Lungs . . . What Smoking Does to Your Lungs . . . The Common Cold — A Healing Crisis . . . Oxygen the Germ-Killer

4. **YOUR DIAPHRAGM — THE KEY TO DEEP BREATHING** 17
   Chest Breathing vs. Diaphragmatic Breathing . . . Internal Massage by Diaphragmatic Action . . . Calming Effect Upon the Nerves

5. **THE IMPORTANCE OF POSTURE** 21
   Correct Posture . . . Wear Loose, Comfortable Clothing . . . Great Singers and Dancers are Deep Breathers . . . Exercise Without Exercise . . . Normalize Your Figure . . . No One Can Breathe for You

6. **PREPARATION FOR SUPER-BRAIN BREATHING** ... 26
   Posture Exercise . . . Exercising the Stomach Muscles . . . Diaphragm Exercise

CHAPTERS

7. **WHAT IS SUPER-BRAIN BREATHING?** 29
   Stimulation of the Pituitary Gland ... Early Morning For Super-Brain Breathing Exercises ... Fresh Air and Warmth Necessary ... Breathe Through the Mouth and Nose Proceed with Caution ... Mental Attitude Important

8. **SUPER-BRAIN BREATHING EXERCISES** 33
   No. 1 — Cleansing Breath ... No. 2 — The Super-Brain Breath ... No. 3 — Super-Kidney Breath ... No. 4 — Blowing the Bowel ... No. 5 — Apex of Lungs ... No. 6 — The Liver Breath ... No. 7 — Heart Strengthener .... Faithfulness Counts

9. **LEARN TO CONTROL YOUR BREATHING** 37
   Evening and Bedtime Routines ... Breathing to Relieve Pain ... Rhythmic Breathing and Walking ... Correct Breathing Makes Exercise a Pleasure ... Tranquilizing Effect on the Nerves ... Relief in Respiratory Ailments

10. **THE PROBLEM OF AIR POLLUTION** 42
    Conserve Your Oxygen with Vitamin E ... Add Vitamin E to Your Diet ... Foods Rich in Vitamin E ... Eating for Oxygen

11. **HEALTH SCHEDULE OF 12 MEALS PER WEEK** 47
    Lunchtime Is Salad Time ... Balanced Variety for Dinner ... Don't Poison Your Body with Foodless Foods and Harmful Drinks ... Don't Use Salt! ... Fast One Day Each Week ... Drink Only Distilled Water

12. **A STRONG MIND IN A STRONG BODY** 53
    Super-Oxygen for Super-Living ... The Advantages of Super-Brain Breathing ... Your Teacher's Final Message of Health

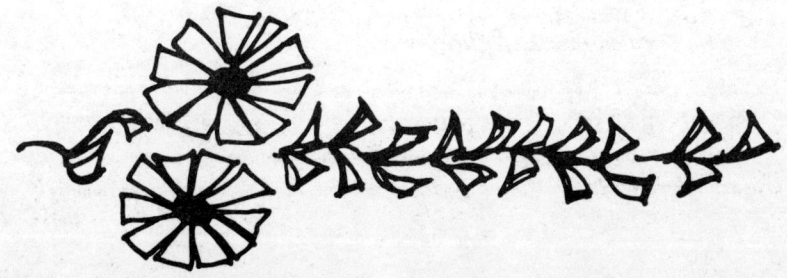

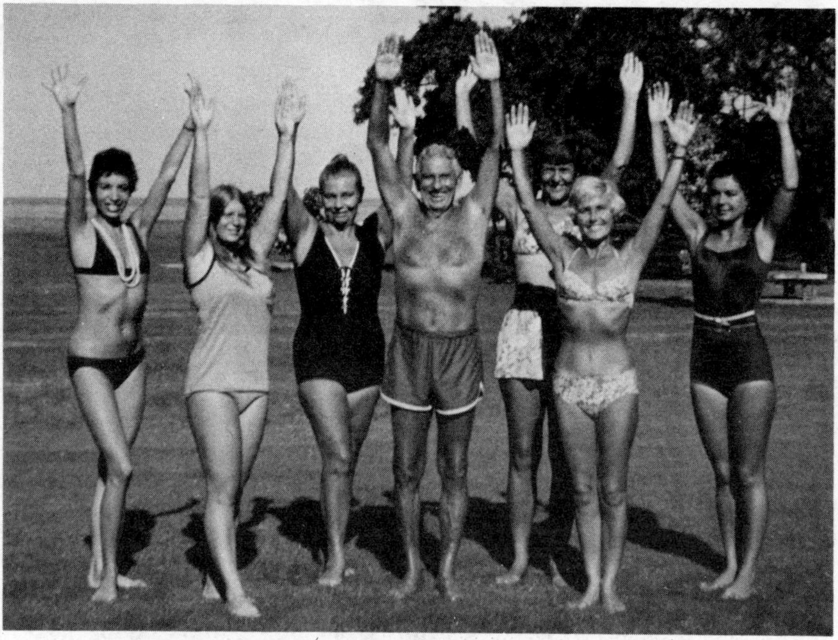

JOIN THE FUN AT THE "LONGER LIFE, HEALTH AND HAPPINESS CLUB" WHEN YOU VISIT HAWAII

Paul and Patricia Bragg and some of their prize members of the "Longer Life, Health and Happiness Club" at their exercise compound at Fort DeRussy, right at Waikiki Beach, Honolulu, Hawaii. Membership is free and open to everyone who wishes to attend any morning Monday through Saturday from 8:30 a.m. to 10:30 a.m. for deep breathing, exercising, meditation, group singing and mini health lectures on how to live a long, healthy life! The group averages 75 to 100 per day. When they are away lecturing they have their leaders carry on until their return. Thousands have visited the club from around the world and then they carry the message of health and happiness to their friends and relatives back home. Paul and Patricia extend an invitation to you and your friends to join the club for health and happiness fellowship with them . . . when you visit Hawaii!

Now I see the secret of the making of the best persons, it is to grow in the open air, and eat and sleep with the earth. —Walt Whitman

---

In health there is liberty. Health is the first of all liberties, happiness gives us the energy which is the basis of health. —Miel

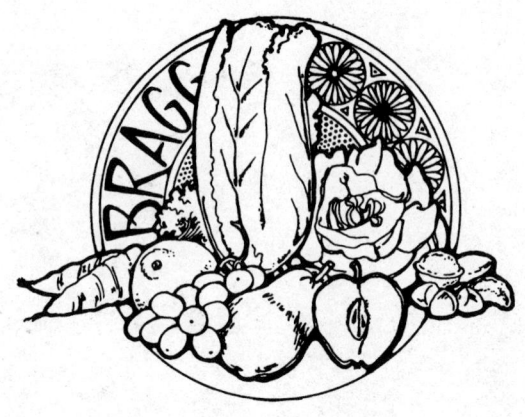

FROM THE AUTHORS

This book was written for YOU. It can be your passport to the Good Life. We Professional Nutritionists join hands in one common objective — a high standard of health for all and many added years to your life. Scientific Nutrition points the way — Nature's Way — the only lasting way to build a body free of degenerative diseases and premature aging. This book teaches you how to work with Nature and not against her. Doctors, dentists, and others who care for the sick, try to repair depleted tissues which too often mend poorly if at all. Many of them praise the spreading of this new scientific message of natural foods and methods for long-lasting health and youthfulness at any age. To speed the spreading of this tremendous message, this book was written.

Statements in this book are recitals of scientific findings, known facts of physiology, biological therapeutics, and reference to ancient writings as they are found. Paul C. Bragg has been practicing the natural methods of living for over 70 years, with highly beneficial results, knowing they are safe and of great value to others, and his daughter Patricia Bragg works with him to carry on the Health Crusade. They make no claims as to what the methods cited in this book will do for one in any given situation, and assume no obligation because of opinions expressed.

No cure for disease is offered in this book. No foods or diets are offered for the treatment or cure of any specific ailment. Nor is it intended as, or to be used as, literature for any food product. Paul C. Bragg and Patricia Bragg express their opinions solely as Public Health Educators, Professional Nutritionists and Teachers.

Certain persons considered experts may disagree with one or more statements in this book, as the same relate to various nutritional recommendations. However, any such statements are considered, nevertheless, to be factual, as based upon long-time experience of Paul C. Bragg and Patricia Bragg in the field of human health.

Chapter 1

Do You Know How To Breathe?

"The breath of life" means exactly what it says. To breathe is to live. Not to breathe is to die. A human being can exist without food for weeks . . . without water for days . . . but without air he cannot exist for even a few minutes.

This fact is so obvious and breathing is so automatic that most people simply take it for granted. *But do you really know how to breathe?* Stop and think about it for a moment. Do you really know how your lungs function? Do you use these marvelous organs to their fullest capacity?

The way you use your lungs controls your health . . . your looks . . . the way you feel . . . your resistance to disease . . . your very life span!

LIVING AT A HIGH RATE OF VIBRATION

As a life extension specialist for well over half a century I have developed techniques for measuring mental and physical energy in humans. Everyone lives at a certain rate of vibration. Unfortunately, very few live at the high rate of which the human body is capable . . . because only a few know how to generate, utilize and replenish their full capacity of energy.

These are the doers. They seem to have inexhaustible vitality and stamina . . . creative power and/or athletic ability of the highest quality. They never seem to tire. They can do mental or physical work without strain, tension or excessive emotion. Everything seems to be easy. Above all, these are happy, contented people who always seem to find the humorous side of life. They are full of personal magnetism. They are enthusiastic beyond the ordinary . . . sociable . . . lovable . . . a pleasure to be with. They have bright and happy dispositions. They are free from "hang ups" and mental blocks. These are the people who enjoy "the good life".

What is their secret? How does one live at a superior rate of vibration?

The answer is really very simple. Such people consume large amounts of oxygen. They breathe deeply and fully . . . utilizing every square inch of their lung capacity.

The more oxygen you can pump into your lungs, the more energy you will have . . . the higher will be your rate of vibration. It is very much like a fire in an open fireplace . . . the more oxygen the fire gets, the brighter it will burn . . . the less it gets, the less fire and more smoke.

LEARN HOW TO INCREASE YOUR ENERGY BY DEEP BREATHING

At age 16, I was officially pronounced a "hopeless case" of tuberculosis . . . but by age 18, I had become a successful athlete. It was during those two years that I was introduced to and cured by the Science of Natural Living . . . to which I have dedicated the rest of my life.

Today I am a great, great-grandfather, to my credit . . . and in any competition requiring energy and stamina, I can outlast most people half and even less than half my age. I hike, jog, swim, climb mountains (I've climbed some of the world's highest), box, wrestle, enjoy competitive games . . . and I can also type for hours without fatigue.

I keep myself in a high rate of mental and physical vibration because I supply my body with the fuel it needs . . . natural live foods . . . and above all, oxygen.

I have helped many people in all walks of life . . . musicians, writers, artists, doctors, lawyers . . . as well as athletes and active sportsmen . . . office workers and housewives . . . to achieve the enjoyment of a superior state of living.

Let me emphasize again that the basic source of super-vibration is knowing how to fill the entire lungs with oxygen. Everyone is born with this capacity, but only a few retain it naturally. Others have developed it, as I am going to show you how to develop it . . . by this system of Super-Brain Breathing.

Whatever your age . . . it is never too early . . . or too late . . . to learn how to increase your energy by the correct method of deep breathing. *Within six months* of faithfully following the breathing exercises which I shall give you in this book . . . you, too, can learn how to fill your lungs with energy-producing oxygen. You will enjoy the thrill of this great natural stimulation . . . a stimulation far more potent than that of any artificial stimulant such as alcohol, coffee, tea, cola drinks or drugs . . . and with no adverse side effects! In fact, the "side effects" of oxygen stimulation add up to the bonus of a longer, fuller lifetime of living.

Life is a pure flame, and we live by an invisible sun within us.
— *Sir Thomas Browne*

LIVING AT A MEDIUM RATE OF VIBRATION

Certain levels of vitality and energy, both mental and physical, are attained by people who live at a medium rate of vibration. While they have a fine capacity for work and play, they are not capable of the sustained effort achieved by those at a high level. Medium-vibration people tire more easily. They lack endurance, particularly under stress. Exhaustion induced by tension and strain forces them to stop and rest.

Such people simply do not get enough vital oxygen to give them that extra something to keep going under physical, mental or emotional pressures. Under extreme pressure they "run out of gas" . . . they don't have what it takes to make that additional effort.

Why? Because they are not using the full capacity of their lungs for energy-producing oxygen . . . they can't get their "second wind". That is the difference between the person who lives in the super-vibration, and those who have achieved only a medium rate of vibration.

VALUE OF THE "SECOND WIND"

At a high rate of vibration . . . consuming your full quota of oxygen . . . you have the capacity for getting your "second wind" . . . and feeling stronger than when you began your effort. That is what makes the great athlete, the great politician, the great statesman, the great professional man or woman, the writer and the go-getter.

When you learn to use the full capacity of your lungs through this system of Super-Brain Breathing, you will experience this wonderful stimulation of the "second wind". Just when you think you have run out of energy and vitality . . . this sudden renewal of strength occurs. It is an experience difficult to describe. To feel that you cannot take another step . . . that your brain power is all gone, your thinking befuddled . . . then suddenly a great surge of energy courses through your entire body, and you feel as fresh and even stronger than when you started. What a tremendous sensation it is! And when you breathe correctly, you experience this "second wind".

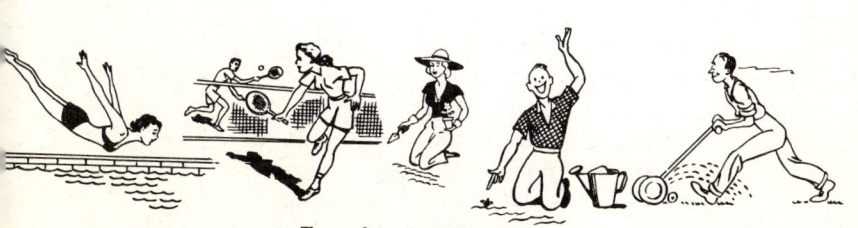

Exercise for Health

MISERY AT A LOW RATE OF VIBRATION

Even the people who live at a medium rate of vibration are in the minority. In our civilized world today, I regret to report, most people are only half-alive . . . they merely exist at a very low rate of physical and mental vibration. This includes all ages . . . from early teens to late eighties (if they live that long).

Research has shown that, in modern civilized countries, only babies use their lungs as Nature intended. All too soon they acquire the unnatural "civilized" habit of shallow breathing. They use only the top part of their lungs. This shallow breathing starves your body of the vital oxygen it must have to be truly alive.

That is why you see so many people . . . from teenagers to oldsters . . . crowding doctors' offices, clinics, sanitariums, convalescent homes, hospitals and cemeteries . . . seeking artificial remedies and palliatives . . . laxatives, pain-killers, tonics, sleeping pills and other drugs.

Oxygen starved people are usually nervous, and suffer from unnecessary worries as well as physical ills. They go to bed tired and get up tired. They suffer from headaches, constipation, indigestion . . . muscular aches and pains, stiff joints . . . aching backs and aching feet . . . aching teeth and sore gums . . . poor eyesight, poor hearing . . . loss of memory . . . sore throats and respiratory ailments such as bronchitis, catarrh and the dread emphysema.

The miseries and loss of healthy bodily functions attributed to "aging" plague these people early in life and take them to an early grave. They suffer and die needlessly . . . simply because they don't know how to breathe correctly! It seems incredible — but it's true.

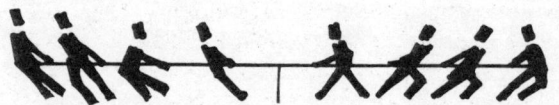

This strange disease of modern life,
With its sick hurry, its divided aims.

— Matthew Arnold

Chapter 2
Oxygen Starvation

Suppose you are very hungry, and sit down to enjoy a well planned, nourishing meal . . . but as soon as you have eaten only one-fourth of the food, someone snatches it away and tells you that you can't have any more. What would you think of the food-snatcher?

Yet this is exactly what you do to yourself when you breathe as most people do, by using only one-fourth to one-third of your lung capacity. You are starving your body much more than if you deprive it of food. You are robbing your body of its most vital nourishment — oxygen.

Without sufficient oxygen, you cannot assimilate the food you eat and drink, no matter how basically nourishing it may be. Oxygen is essential to the process of ionization, or the breaking up of food molecules into nutritious materials suitable for the body's needs.

Without sufficient oxygen, your bloodstream becomes saturated with poisonous carbon dioxide and other toxic wastes . . . and transports these throughout your system (collecting more enroute) . . . thus suffocating the cells of your body . . . instead of rejuvenating them with life-giving oxygen.

Your brain, which requires three times more oxygen than the rest of your body, suffers first. According to Philip Rice, M.D., a morphologist who has worked all his life with delinquent children. **55% delinquency in minors can be attributed to oxygen starvation** as a result of shallow breathing and lack of fresh air. Educators who are alarmed about the decrease in the average I.Q. would do well to consider this factor. Tests and analyses are not brain food . . . oxygen is.

You can make a simple demonstration by lighting two candles and placing them side by side, a few inches apart. Now partially cover one candle with a glass . . . watch how much smaller and paler this flame becomes. If you cover the candle completely with the glass, the flame will go out in a few seconds. That is what happens in your body when you deprive it of oxygen.

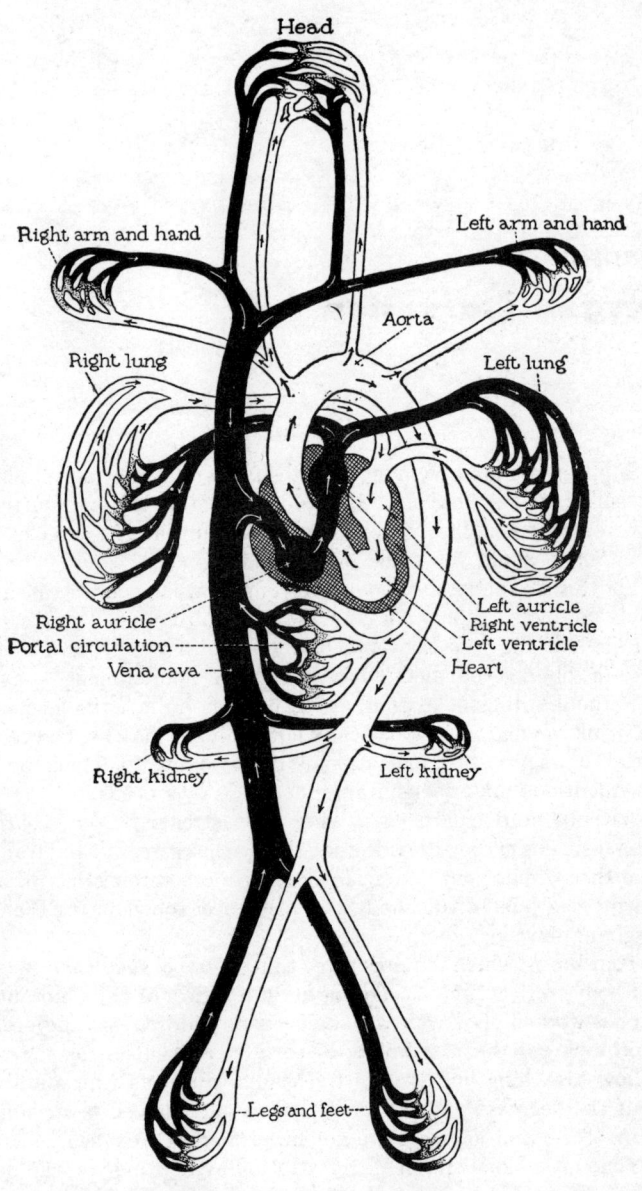

THE HEART AND BLOOD-VESSEL SYSTEM. The diagram shows the cycle from right heart through the lungs, to the left heart, then through the system back to the right heart. Note that all the blood from the digestive system goes through the portal veins; i.e., through the liver.

OXYGEN POWERS THE HUMAN MACHINE

The human body is a marvelous and intricate mechanism for the production of mental and physical energy. Oxygen is the power source by which this mechanism operates. Your body begins to function with your first breath and continues until your last. How well it functions depends on how well you supply it with oxygen power.

As in any heat or combustion engine, oxygen is essential to the production of energy in your body. Every flame consists of the union of oxygen with other elements. The gasoline that fuels your car, the natural gas or coal in heater or furnace, the wood in a fireplace or stove ...all contain latent energy...but it cannot be released to produce heat or power until its elements are broken down and united with oxygen.

In the human body this process is called metabolism. The food you eat contains latent energy, but it is of absolutely no use to you without oxygen. In determining the general health of the human body a test is made of the basal metabolism, the rate being determined by measure of the oxygen utilized while the body is in a resting state.

As long as you live, the body mechanism operates continuously. Even when you are asleep, your lungs and heart, your kidneys, liver and other major organs, your circulatory and nervous systems must continue to function. The amount of energy you need depends, of course, upon your activities, mental as well as physical. And the release of the energy you need depends upon your intake of oxygen.

OXYGEN CARRIED BY THE BLOODSTREAM

Every one of the 40 trillion cells in your body demands a continuous flow of life-giving oxygen in order to stay alive, do its job, and remain healthy. This oxygen supply is carried in your bloodstream by the red blood cells, or red corpuscles . . . and there are millions of these red cells in every drop of blood.

The blood circulates in a network of 100,000 miles of blood vessels that reach every cell in the body, from those of the heart itself to the top of the scalp and the tips of the fingers and toes. In the average individual there are 6 to 8 quarts of blood circulating in this vast network.

During rest or inactivity the blood makes one round trip per minute. During activity or exercise, however, it may make as many as 8 or 9 round trips per minute in order to supply the necessary fuel and oxygen for increased energy, and remove the burnt-out wastes.

The blood vessels which carry the blood from the heart are known as arteries. Those which return the blood to the heart are called veins. Both vary greatly in size, just like the streamlets and brooks and creeks which flow into a river, which may then join a larger river.

The smallest of both the arteries and the veins are called capillaries . . . so tiny that most are visible only under a microscope. It is through these capillaries that the last of the food and oxygen is given off and the transfer is made into the veins, which carry the oxygen-depleted blood and toxic wastes back to the heart for purification. Enroute to the heart most of the water soluble wastes are transferred to the kidneys for elimination from the body through the urine.

The poisonous carbon dioxide gas, a major residue of energizing oxidation, is brought back to the heart to be expelled through the lungs.

PURIFICATION OF THE BLOOD

The carbon dioxide collected from all parts of the body gives the blood a bluish color when it is returned through the veins to the heart. There it enters the right auricle, or upper chamber of the right side of the heart. When this is filled, the valve into the right ventricle, or lower chamber, opens to fill it, then closes as the strong muscles of the ventricle contract and send the blood into the lungs.

Through the capillary network of the lung sacs, the blood discharges its load of carbon dioxide . . . turns a bright red again as it absorbs the life-giving oxygen . . . and returns immediately to the left auricle of the heart. From there it goes into the left ventricle by similar valve action, and is pumped vigorously into the body's largest artery, the aorta, from which it is distributed through the vast arterial network throughout the rest of the body . . . bringing the vital oxygen and accompanying nutrients to every cell.

It is the shorter or "lesser" circulation, as it is called . . . from the heart to the lungs and back . . . that is so vital to purify the bloodstream. If the lungs are only partially filled with air, only that part of the bloodstream can be cleansed. The blood which passes through the capillaries of empty air sacs cannot get rid of its carbon dioxide wastes and cannot pick up oxygen. So, instead of carrying a full quota of life-giving oxygen back to the cells of the body, the bloodstream returns with a mixture of fresh oxygen and a residue of toxic poisons. As this process continues, the proportion of toxic carbon dioxide increases.

This is what happens when you do not breathe fully and deeply. When your breathing is shallow, you do not change the air at the base of your lungs, where two-thirds of the lung capacity is located. When you return impure blood to the rest of your body, the ill effects are compounded because the blood itself cannot perform its proper functions.

Most men employ the first part of life to make the other part miserable.
— La Bruyère

SHALLOW BREATHERS POISON THEMSELVES

Loaded with poisonous wastes, the blood has difficulty in transporting the comparatively small amount of oxygen which it does absorb . . . nor can it carry the necessary nourishment from food. The breaking down of food molecules into digestible elements is impaired . . . all bodily functions are slowed down without an adequate oxygen supply.

The organs of elimination are overworked . . . and underfed. But the accumulating wastes must go somewhere. Some are discharged by overloading the sweat glands, producing unpleasant body odors. Other toxic wastes are deposited as heavy mucus in the sinus cavities, lungs and bronchial tubes . . . along the passages of the ears, eyes, nose and throat . . . and along the digestive tract. Hardened wastes are deposited in the movable joints and spine, where pressure on nerves signals the warning of pain. (Pain is Nature's alarm that something is seriously wrong . . . it should be heeded by corrective action . . . not silenced by drugs.)

By robbing their bodies of vital oxygen, shallow breathers are actually poisoning themselves . . . inflicting tortures upon their bodies while committing slow suicide. They are suffering from autointoxication, or self-poisoning . . . dying in their own body poisons.

If someone else deliberately tried to force you to kill yourself in this manner, what would you do? You'd fight back, wouldn't you? In defiance, you would breathe deeply and fully . . . cleansing your blood . . purifying your entire system . . . making your body tingle with life and energy.

Why not do it now?

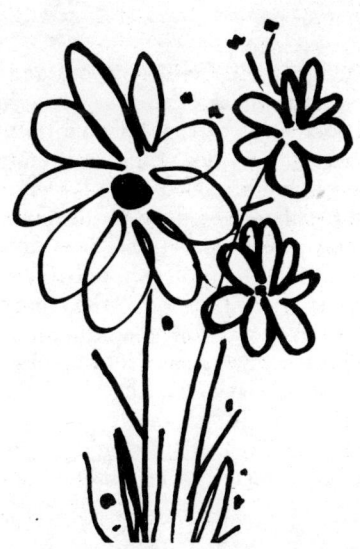

Chapter 3

The Way You Breathe Is The Way You Live

When you breathe deeply and fully . . . you live deeply and fully.

When a generous flow of oxygen is being pumped into your body, every cell comes alive. The four main "motors" of the body . . . the heart, the lungs . . . the liver and the kidneys . . . operate at peak performance. Your bloodstream purifies itself . . . cleanses every part of the body and transports the toxic wastes to be eliminated as Nature planned . . . and carries fuel-food and vital oxygen to every cell.

Your muscles, tendons and joints function smoothly. Your flesh becomes firm and resilient . . . your skin clear and glowing . . . your hair lustruous. You radiate health and wellbeing.

Your brain becomes alert . . . your nervous system functions perfectly. You are free from tension and strain . . . you withstand stresses and pressures with ease.

Emotions are under control. You feel joyous and exuberant. When negative emotions try to intrude . . . such as anger, hate, jealousy, fear or grief . . . they are expelled by concentrated deep breathing.

The deep breather enjoys peace of mind, serenity and tranquility. All the Great Masters in India teach deep, full breathing as the first essential for higher spiritual development. You get perfect concentration in meditation by long, slow, deep breaths. Deep breathing stimulates the higher brain cells. The more deeply and fully you breathe, the greater is your power of concentration . . . the more fully your creative power will assert itself. You develop greater extra sensory perception.

The person who breathes deeply and fully thinks clearly . . . oxygen stimulates logic and intelligence. You become master of your entire body. Deep, full breathing will constantly rejuvenate your body to a higher vibration of living. The more fully and deeply you breathe, the farther you will travel to higher levels on the physical, mental and spiritual planes.

YOUR MARVELOUS LUNGS

Every living thing breathes. Plants breathe through pores in their leaves. In the marvelous balance of Nature, plants breathe in carbon dioxide and give off oxygen ... while animals inhale oxygen and exhale carbon dioxide. In natural balance, both thrive. But man has played havoc with this natural balance by destroying forests, covering grass with pavements ... and to air already thus polluted by an excess of carbon dioxide, he continues to add more pollutants from motorized traffic and industry. Wildlife (the remainder which has survived slaughter by man) suffocates in such atmosphere. Fish die in polluted waters. How long can man survive in the midst of the environmental poisons which he creates has become a question of concern.

Every animal extracts oxygen from the medium in which it lives. Through their gills fish extract oxygen from water ($H2O$). Insects get it from the air through alveoli or air cells in individual openings set in segments of their bodies. Worms and other invertebrates breathe through their skin pores.

Vertebrate animals (those with a spinal column) including man evolved the wonderful mechanism of the lungs. The mechanical equivalent would be a pair of bellows ... but the lungs are far more intricate and adaptable.

Composed of spongy, porous tissue, the lungs are a pair of concial shaped organs which, with the heart in the center, occupy the thoracic cavity or chest ... the upper half of the human torso, protected by the rib cage. The apex of each lung reaches just above the collar bone ... the base, or lower lobes, extending to the waistline.

The lungs are composed of some 800 million alveoli, air cells or sacs, of elastic tissue which can expand or contract like tiny balloons. If these little air sacs were flattened out and laid side by side, the flattened alveoli would cover an area of 100 square yards.

Tiny capillaries (blood vessels) thread the elastic walls of each of the hundreds of millions of air sacs ... and it is through these that the blood passes to discharge its load of poisonous carbon dioxide and absorb the life-giving oxygen. This cleansing in the body's 6 quarts of blood (average man) must be performed from *1 to 9 times a minute,* depending upon activity from rest to running.

Air inhaled through the nose and/or mouth reaches the alveoli through an intricate system of tubes, beginning with the large trachea, or windpipe, which is kept rigid by rings of cartilage in its walls. The trachea extends through the neck into the chest, where it divides into two branches, or bronchi, one leading into each lung. The bonchi divide into a number of smaller and smaller branches to reach every air sac.

Each lung is enveloped in a protective elastic membrane, the pleura, whose inner layer is attached to the lung ... and whose outer layer forms the lining of the thoracic cavity, inside the rib cage. Although one

PATH OF BREATH

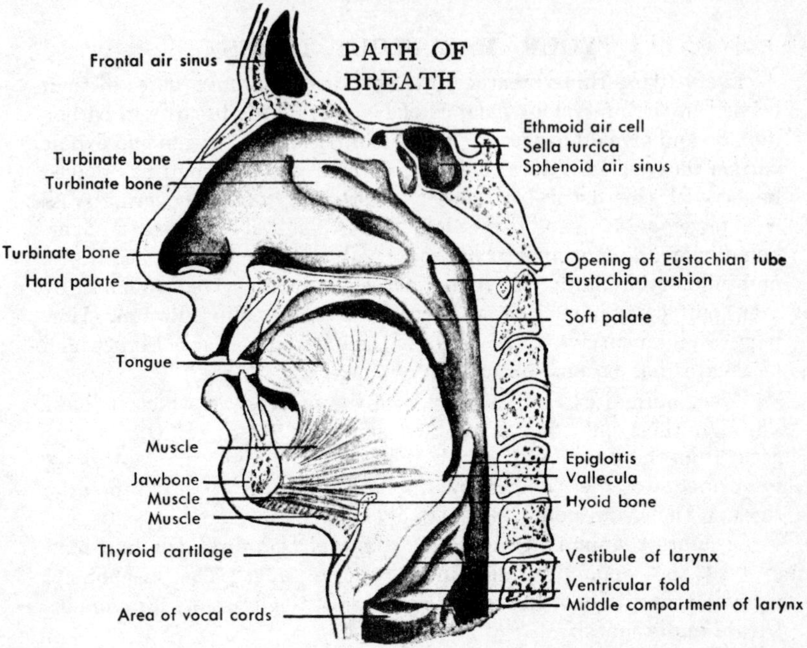

- Frontal air sinus
- Turbinate bone
- Turbinate bone
- Turbinate bone
- Hard palate
- Tongue
- Muscle
- Jawbone
- Muscle
- Muscle
- Thyroid cartilage
- Area of vocal cords
- Ethmoid air cell
- Sella turcica
- Sphenoid air sinus
- Opening of Eustachian tube
- Eustachian cushion
- Soft palate
- Epiglottis
- Vallecula
- Hyoid bone
- Vestibule of larynx
- Ventricular fold
- Middle compartment of larynx

THE LOWER RESPIRATORY SYSTEM

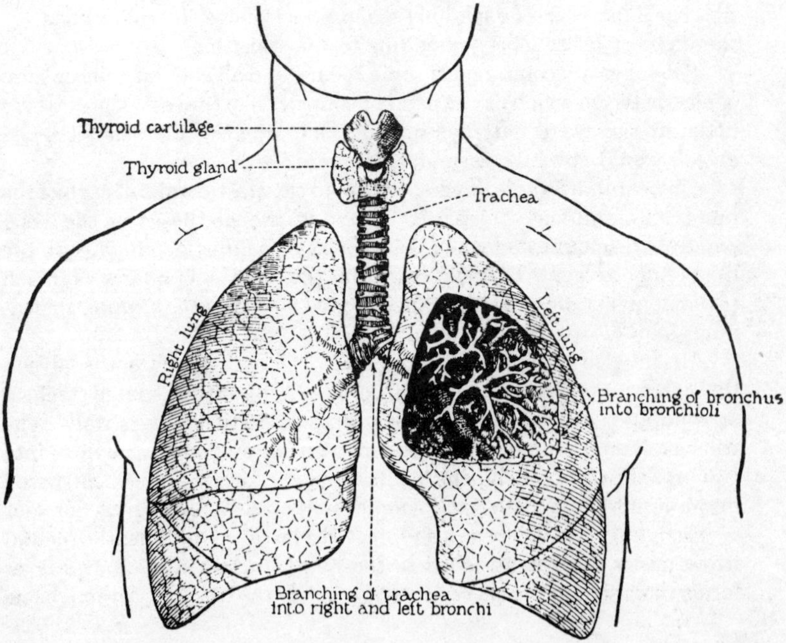

- Thyroid cartilage
- Thyroid gland
- Trachea
- Right lung
- Left lung
- Branching of bronchus into bronchioli
- Branching of trachea into right and left bronchi

end of each rib is attached to the spinal column, the front of the rib cage is open, allowing for expansion and contraction of the lungs.

When you breathe deeply, filling every air sac, your thoracic cavity expands as your lungs fill to capacity with some 6 to 10 pints of air (depending on body build and size), occupying approximately 200 to over 300 cubic inches.

And this marvelous mechanism is yours for free! You are born with it. It functions without conscious effort . . . yet without it, you could not exist.

No invention of man, however ingenious, can equal the human breathing apparatus. The "iron lung" is misnamed . . . lifesaver that it is, it is merely a cumbersome outside contraption to replace paralyzed muscles . . . to enable those marvelous human lungs to function.

Perhaps if human beings had to pay some fabulous price for their lungs, they would use them to full capacity all the time. But did you ever stop to think of the price you pay for *not* using them? Remember, we are always "only one breath away from death"!

WHAT SMOKING DOES TO YOUR LUNGS

When we are born, our lungs are shiny and new, fresh and clean, rose-pink in color. If we could live in a dust-free atmosphere and breathe correctly all our lives, our lungs would remain "as good as new" throughout a lifetime of use.

But what most lungs get is abuse. Some of this comes from external causes. The lungs are the only organ of the body which is directly affected by conditions external to it . . . i.e., the air we breathe. Nature has provided protection against a normal amount of dust contamination . . . with tiny hairs in the nose to serve as filters . . . moist mucus in the passages leading to the lungs to trap dust particles to be expelled through nose or mouth. The tonsils trap a number of germs . . . and the lungs protect themselves remarkably well through oxygenation and by discharge of toxins into the blood for elimination via the kidneys, as well as their own expelling of carbon dioxide.

However, the conditions under which most civilized humans live today are unnatural. Certainly there is an abnormal amount of pollutants in the air we breathe, especially in urban areas. Our lungs are often overloaded with more contaminants than they can handle, and these are passed along into the bloodstream and to other parts of the body. The lungs of a modern city dweller become brownish from oil smog or gray from coal soot . . . and even in farming country, the lungs must contend with excess dust and poisonous pesticides.

With all these handicaps to overcome, it seems incredible that anyone would deliberately further endanger the health of the lungs . . . and the entire body . . . by smoking!

To begin with, *nicotine* is a poisonous drug. One of its effects, directly related to lung function, is *constriction of the capillaries* . . . impairing the flow of blood through the walls of the air sacs. Tobacco also *neutralizes Vitamin C*, which is active in preventing hemorrhaging of the capillaries.

The air sacs are further damaged by tobacco tars and carbon particles that lodge in the walls of these balloon-like cells . . . causing them to lose their elasticity . . . and finally to break down altogether. The destruction of the air sacs is *the dread emphysema*, the killer disease which slowly smothers its victim from within.

So much has been said and written about *lung cancer* as a result of smoking that I do not need to repeat it here. I will merely remind you that medical and clinical evidence overwhelmingly proves the far greater incidence of cancer of the lungs, larynx and pharynx, esophagus and oral cavity among heavy smokers.

Smoking also introduces two other deadly poisons into the body, *arsenic* and *carbon monoxide.*

Of course, if you insist upon committing suicide by smoking, no one can stop you. But if you really want to save your lungs, your health and your life . . . yet consider it "impossible" to stop smoking . . . all I can say is, "Who controls your body — the tobacco or you?" Flesh is dumb. It has no intelligence. You must control the body with the mind. In my lecture work throughout the world I have had health students in my classes who have smoked for as long as 50 years . . . and they stopped without tapering off. They made up their minds to stop smoking at once . . . and they did. So can you!

(NOTE: For the effect of smoking on the heart, see my book, *"How to Keep the Heart Healthy and Fit".)*

Here's a tip from a writer friend of mine, who over the years had acquired the bad habit of lighting a cigarette whenever she paused in her writing to correlate the next sequence of thought. She finally realized that the reason she did this was because her brain was calling for more oxygen and what she actually needed and wanted was a deep breath . . . but she was inhaling smoke instead of oxygen . . . thus defeating her purpose. Instead of being refreshed, she became more tired.

"When it dawned on me what I was doing, I felt like a complete fool," she wrote me. "Now, instead of a cigarette, I take a full, deep breath . . . and my thoughts come faster and more clearly than ever."

Try it! When you reach for a cigarette (or cigar or pipe) . . . stop! Take a long, slow deep breath, filling every air sac in your lungs . . . hold it, while your red blood cells become re-oxygenated . . . then exhale slowly and completely, emptying every bit of poisonous carbon dioxide from your lungs. You will feel a new surge of energy from the top of your scalp to the soles of your feet . . . a relaxing and at the same time rejuvenating sensation which you will never get from tobacco or any other artifical stimulant!

The surest way to rid yourself of a bad habit is to replace it with a good one. There could be no greater benefit to your life and health than to replace smoking by deep breathing!

THE COMMON COLD — A HEALING CRISIS

Every day in wintertime some 30 million Americans are suffering with "a bad cold". Adults average 5 to 6 colds per season, children and teenagers as high as 6 to 12.

Are these colds necessary? How do people "catch cold"? What causes the common cold? Medical science has learned how to control many diseases that are far more serious, but remains baffled by this "minor infection". Is the culprit an unfilterable virus, as has been suggested? Is it brought on by sitting in a draught, getting chilled, getting one's feet wet?

There are many theories. But there seems to be only one sure fact... people who are in perfect health don't "catch cold". I spent a year living in the Arctic country among the Eskimos. I never had a cold, and neither did they. I have had the same experience in the South Seas . . . in the Balkans . . . among nomads of the Middle East and primitive tribes of Africa. The common factor among all these peoples is that they breathe pure air, eat natural foods, and get plenty of exercise and sleep.

By following this same same basic regime, I remain free of colds even in the midst of civilization.

Based on my own research, I believe that the "common cold" is Nature's method of detoxifying the body. Most humans who exist on the average, devitalized foods of civilization and are shallow breathers accumulate in their bodies a "cesspool" of uneliminated toxins.

When these accumulated poisons reach a point beyond the toxic tolerance of the body, the natural vital forces of the body set up a healing crisis. A rise in body temperature, or fever, is induced to burn up many toxic poisons . . . while others are eliminated by a heavy discharge of mucus from the nose, mouth and throat. If the toxic overload is very heavy, there will also be a discharge of mucus from the bowels and diarrhea.

Instead of being alarmed, be grateful that your natural vital forces are strong enough to take command and get rid of the toxic trash you have accumulated. Don't try to block this natural process with drugs. Instead, work with Nature. Rest and fast. Drink fruit and vegetable juices or herb teas and steam distilled water . . . but take nothing else into your stomach during this crisis period. Breathe deeply and fully to supply your body with that great purifier, oxygen.

Your body is a self-healing organism . . . and it will fight for its life against a great deal of abuse. When you follow Nature's laws . . . as I have done for some 75 years . . . you will never be ill. You will have a painless, tireless, ageless body.

If you "catch cold" remember you are passing through a natural healing crisis . . . and heed the warning. Mother Nature is saying to you, "You have allowed your body to become poisoned with toxic wastes. Work with me now to cleanse your system of these poisons . . . and once this crisis is passed, continue to work with me and keep it clean by following my laws of natural living."

OXYGEN THE GERM-KILLER

So often someone tells me that he/she has just had a bad case of "flu". When I ask where they think they got the "flu", they usually parrot the old broken record, "Oh, don't you know that the flu is going around?"

So I play coy and ask, "Where will I find it? I would like to meet some flu germs."

They stare at me in utter amazement.

To help them out of their mental confusion, I then explain that when you live on a diet of natural foods . . . that is, foods free from all refining, processing and chemical additives . . . and breathe fully and deeply, you build a powerful immunity against all virus and germs.

No germ, for example, can live in pure, freshly squeezed orange juice, because there is nothing in pure orange juice for it to feed on. All germs, regardless of their names, are scavengers . . . they feed on decaying matter.

It is my personal opinion, based on my own experience and research, that a natural immunity against infectious diseases is based upon a diet of 100% whole, natural foods . . . plus a tremendous amount of pure oxygen being pumped into the body by vigorous breathing exercises, as outlined in this book.

Oxygen is the great purifier, the great natural cleanser. Oxygen is not only the energizing factor which makes it possible for the body to eliminate the putrefactive matter on which germs thrive . . . it also exterminates the germs themselves.

The more oxygen you pump into your body, the freer you will be of any sort of infection.

When we practice Super-Brain Breathing, we increase our cardiovascular respiratory power . . . that is, we purify and energize our bloodstream so that it carries purifying, vitalizing oxygen to the heart and other organs and to every cell in the body.

The human body has one ability not possesed by any machine—the ability to repair itself.
—George E. Crile, Jr., M.D.

Chapter 4

Your Diaphragm —
The Key To Deep Breathing

What is the secret of deep breathing? How do you draw in air to the very base of your lungs? Certainly not by merely sniffing it in through your nose . . . nor by gaping it in with a yawn through your mouth.

The natural method of deep breathing . . . the way babies breathe ... is by using the diaphragm to create suction that pulls the air into the lungs. Air may enter the body through either the nose or the mouth, but the force which draws it in to fill the air sacs of the lungs to capacity is the muscular action of the diaphragm.

The diaphragm is a dome-shaped sheet of strong muscle fibers that separates the thoracic (upper) half of your body containing the heart and lungs, from the abdominal (lower) cavity which houses the organs of digestion and elimination. It stretches from the sternum (breastbone) in front across the bottom of the ribs to the backbone.

When the diaphragm expands and flattens moving downward, it produces suction within the chest cavity which causes an inflow of air into the lungs (inhalation). When the diaphragm relaxes and rises, air is forced out of the lungs (exhalation). Both operations are of equal importance . . . inhalation to bring in life-giving oxygen . . . exhalation to expel every bit of poisonous carbon dioxide.

CHEST BREATHING VERSUS DIAPHRAGMATIC BREATHING

A great deal is often made about "chest expansion" . . . the number of inches which the chest expands from a collapsed or relaxed position after exhalation to that when the lungs are filled with air.

Chest breathing is breathing which results from the movement of the rib section of the trunk, especially the upper section of the chest. During inhalation the chest expands (becomes larger), and during exhalation it relaxes (becomes smaller). This form of breathing, especially when performed to the limit of inhalation and exhalation, is an excellent form of internal exercise, developing the size of the chest which is beneficial in many ways. However, the man with a big chest is not any better off than the man with an average size lung box, if the latter uses his breathing organs so as to get oxygen throughout his body.

Chest breathing is naturally employed by the body only during strenuous exertion. It might be termed a form of "forced breathing", just as a forced draught may be applied to a boiler in case great steam pressure is needed. It is an emergency measure.

Unfortunately, as mentioned previously, most people rob themselves of oxygen by breathing with only a minimum use of the top of the chest.

Diaphragmatic breathing, as noted, is the natural method for which the human body was designed. When the diaphragm expands, it not only expands the chest cavity and draws air into the lungs . . . it also expands the abdominal cavity, not for the purpose of drawing in air, but for stretching the abdominal muscles and organs. When the diaphragm relaxes, it not only expels air from the lungs and further exercises the rib muscles . . . but it also tightens the abdominal muscles and compresses the organs.

INTERNAL MASSAGE BY DIAPHRAGMATIC ACTION

The effect of the expansion and relaxation of the diaphragm on the muscles and organs of the abdomen is highly beneficial.

From the long point of view of evolution, the erect posture of man is relatively recent. To combat the pull of gravity and hold the abdominal organs in place, our abdominal muscles need all the exercise we can give them. Correct, natural diaphragmatic breathing accomplishes this.

More than that, it provides important massage for the liver, stomach, intestines, kidneys, gall bladder, spleen and pancreas . . . stimulating the circulation of the blood through these vital organs and aiding them in performing their functions so essential to our health.

In fact, the dual action of the diaphragm . . . affecting both the upper thoracic organs (heart and lungs) and the lower abdominal organs . . . is a vital factor in blood circulation, especially in the return of the blood through the veins to the heart.

The forceful pumping thrust of the heart muscles sends the blood coursing through the arteries . . . but this force is almost spent by the time the bloodstream has dispensed oxygen and nutrients and collected wastes, and is ready to return to the heart through the veins. The return trip is dependent upon body movements . . . contraction of the muscles and muscular walls of the viscera (the internal organs of the body, especially those contained within the abdominal and thoracic cavities),

MECHANICS OF BREATHING

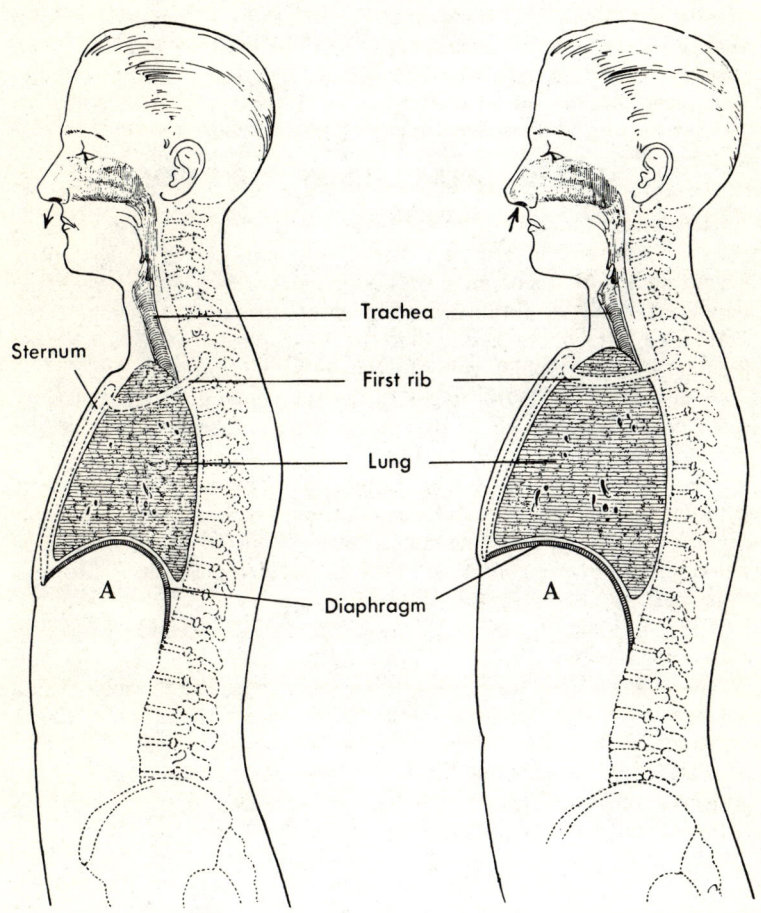

EXHALATION   INHALATION

The mechanics of breathing showing the position of the diaphragm and ribs at expiration and at inspiration.

which squeeze or push the blood through valves set in the veins to guide the bloodstream back to the heart. The rhymthic massage of the abdominal organs by the respiratory muscles plays a vital role in this venous circulation.

Diaphragmatic breathing also *stimulates peristalsis*, a worm-like motion of the intestines, which promotes digestion and the elimination of solid and semi-solid toxic wastes. I know hundreds of cases in which a change from chest to diaphragmatic breathing helped to correct long standing conditions of chronic constipation, gas, heartburn, indigestion, liver troubles, etc.

CALMING EFFECT UPON THE NERVES

The *solar plexus*, the "power house" of the body . . . a network of ganglia (independent groups of nerve cells) and nerves which control every important vital organ in the abdominal cavity . . . is located in the very center of the diaphragm. The more stimulation you give the diaphragm, the more circulation the solar plexus receives and the greater the nerve energy going to your vital organs.

The important *pneumo-gastric nerve (pneumo*, lungs; *gastro*, stomach) passes through the diaphragm and is also greatly benefited by diaphragmatic action.

The tranquilizing rhythm of diaphragmatic breathing, as well as its stimulation of circulation and general rejuvenating effect, has a calming effect upon the entire nervous system. It breaks up the paralyzing nerve tension so often observed in people with super-sensitive and even deranged nerves.

(For more details about the beneficial effects of deep breathing on the nerves, see my book, *"Building A Powerful Nerve Force".)*

According to the teaching of yoga, such deep, rhythmic breathing attunes one to the "rhythm of the universe" . . . in other words, in rhythmic harmony with Nature. "Prana", the yoga word for "breath", also embodies the meaning absolute energy or vital cosmic energy . . . which, according to yoga, is stored in the solar plexus when we draw in a surplus through correct diaphragmatic breathing.

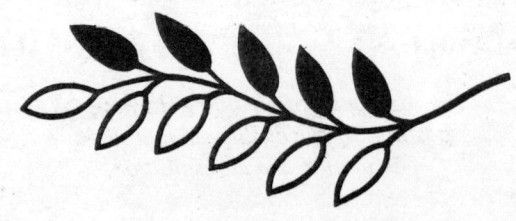

Chapter 5

The Importance of Posture

Today's human, from skeleton to skin, is built to stand erect, sit erect, and walk erect. Now that we have reviewed the way your breathing apparatus operates, you can readily see how essential correct posture is to correct breathing. When you slump, you squeeze your lungs (and other organs, as well) into a cramped position and seriously limit the operation of your diaphragm. You make yourself into a shallow breather, able only to use the top of your lungs. When you sit bent over a desk, at study or work, you rob your body of oxygen, impair circulation, hamper the functions of all vital organs, stretch your muscles and bones into unnatural positions . . . and then wonder why you become so fatigued! You probably also cross your legs, further blocking the circulation to that part of your body and preparing the way for broken capillaries and varicose veins.

The chances are that you maintain the same poor posture when on your feet, standing or walking with shoulders and head drooping or neck outthrust. Nor do you improve matters by going to the opposite extreme. You distort your body and all its components by an exaggerated reversal . . . i.e., thrusting your shoulders and hips back and sticking out your stomach.

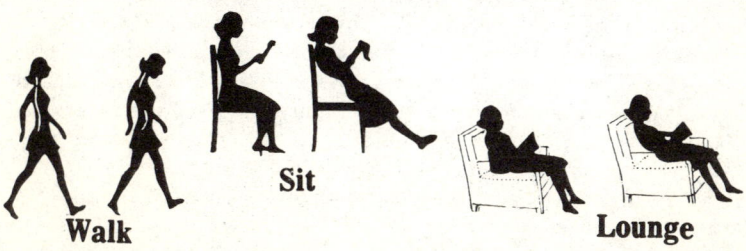

CORRECT POSTURE

Don't make an "S" of your body in either direction. For correct posture, align your body with an imaginary plumb line from the center of the top of your head through the center of your pelvis to midway between the arches of your feet. Stand up with your feet parallel, about six inches apart. Pull your abdomen up out of your hips . . . your chest up out of your abdomen . . . and your neck up out of your chest. Set your shoulders back easily and comfortably. Stand tall . . . but relaxed. Don't you feel a lot better? Take a look in your mirror and see how much better you look, too!

When you sit, keep your trunk in the same position. Sit on your hips, with your feet flat on the floor or ankles lightly crossed. You can work for hours at your desk in this position without fatigue, stopping every now and then for a good stretch. Hold the same basic posture when you walk, letting your arms swing naturally in rhythm with your stride.

WEAR LOOSE, COMFORTABLE CLOTHING

Now don't spoil it all with tight clothing! Tight belts, tight collars, tight foundation garments, tight garters, tight shoes . . . all such restrictive clothing hampers breathing, blood circulation and all major organs. It also throws your body off balance and out of alignment, tight shoes especially . . . and jangles your nerves.

The sloppy clothes of teenagers, worn as an outward show of rebellion against the vogue of "plastic people", indicate an unconscious but natural rebellion of the human body against restrictive clothing. The general overall trend toward comfortable sports clothes is healthy.

I pride myself on being able to take the coldest kind of weather with a small amount of clothing. I never wear a hat, or undershirt, nor do I sleep with anything on. I sleep in the raw. And I swim in all parts of the world in all kinds of weather.

On several occasions the noted Dr. Robert Jackson and I had great sport breaking the ice and swimming with the Boston Brownies of the famous "L" Street Bath House in Boston, Massachusetts. Here you find some of the finest specimens of physical manhood in the world . . . including men in their sixties, seventies and even eighties. The same is true of the Polar Bears in New York City, the boys at Montrose Beach in Chicago and at Bradford Beach in Milwaukee. All these hearty men . . . who enjoy swimming in ice cold water . . . are deep and full breathers. Many of them are my students to whom I have taught my System of Super-Brain Breathing. When you know Super-Brain Breathing, you love to swim in ice cold water.

Now I do not recommend that everyone jump into ice cold water! Let's leave that to the Paul Braggs and other people who have built a body with perfect thermostatic control. I just wanted to give you an idea of how much power you can develop in the body when you are filled with oxygen at all times. There is no limit to your powers of resistance. There is no feeling of wellbeing as great as when every cell in the body is filled with life-giving oxygen.

GREAT SINGERS AND DANCERS ARE DEEP BREATHERS

Breath control . . . by deep diaphragmatic breathing . . . comes first, last and always with the professional singer. Without benefit of loudspeakers, the voices of the great opera singers have filled the auditoriums of the Metropolitan, La Scala and other famous opera houses throughout the world. What diaphragms they had! Look at the body build of these men and women . . . the beautiful, perfect posture . . . the superior development of the torso, with tremendous lung capacity. Listen to the recordings of Caruso, the greatest known voice of all time . . . hear the perfect control, from the softest pure note to the swell of a great crescendo.

Study the lives of these people . . . and you will find that they lived and are living in perfect health . . . filled with energy and charm, regardless of age . . . and they are remarkably long-lived.

The same is true of great dancers. Ruth St. Denis and Ted Shawn thrilled audiences throughout their lifetimes, from their teens into their seventies. Deep diaphragmatic breathing was the key to the tremendous energy and muscular control demanded by their spectacular dances . . . and also the key to their long, healthy, radiant lives.

Deep diaphragmatic breathing is basic in the rigorous training of the Ballet Russe, Sadlers Wells Ballet and all the famous ballet companies . . . as well as the Fred Astaire type of dancers and the rollicking Rockettes of New York's Rockefeller Center. These people are healthy and long-lived, retaining perpetual youthfulness.

While I was in North Africa I was amazed at the beauty, strength and endurance of their native dancers. Their secret, too, was the excellent development of the diaphragm in breathing. Through its action in drawing in large quantities of fresh air and throwing out waste material, these girls have an exquisite complexion and skin, sparkling eyes, remarkable grace and suppleness.

So you aren't a singer or dancer? Is that any reason why you shouldn't enjoy good health and a good life? Without having to undergo the rigorous training of a professional performer, you can profit by their key secrets . . . deep diaphragmatic breathing, regular exercise, and a healthful, natural diet.

EXERCISE WITHOUT EXERCISE

Begin with correct posture. This is essential before you can breathe correctly.

Whenever you are walking, standing or sitting, always lift up the chest and diaphragm. By doing this, you will constantly be using the most important muscles of the body.

The key to firm muscles all over the body is good posture. Remember, poor posture puts your heart, lungs and all your "working machinery" into a vise-like grip which impairs circulation and efficiency. Keep saying to yourself, "I must lift up the chest and diaphragm." In that way you will be exercising all your waking hours. And you will acquire a strength and tone to the muscles that no regular exercise period can give you.

There is nothing so important to good health, vitality and the prolongation of life as correct posture. Keep a straight line from the chin to the toes when standing. Don't slump in your chair when sitting. Keep the head, chest and diaphragm held up high. It may tire you at first, because most people have let themselves get into poor posture habits. But once you give strength and tone to the many muscles which control good posture, you will find yourself more relaxed and free from fatigue.

Which One Are You?

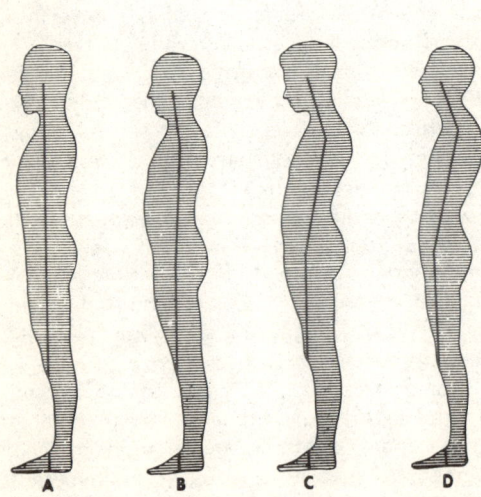

(A) Good: head, trunk, and thigh in straight line; chest high and forward; abdomen flat; back curves normal. (B) Fair: head forward; abdomen prominent; exaggerated curve in upper back; slightly hollow back. (C) Poor: relaxed (fatigue) posture; head forward; abdomen relaxed; shoulder blades prominent; hollow back. (D) Very poor: head forward badly; very exaggerated curve in upper back; abdomen relaxed; chest flat-sloping; hollow back.

NORMALIZE YOUR FIGURE

Fat or thin . . . pot-belly or sway-back . . . you can actually build a new body and a normal figure by correct posture and breathing exercises. All deep breathing exercises are building exercises, because oxygen is the invisible food for the body . . . and causes perfect assimilation of other foods. The very same exercises will build up a person who is underweight . . . and trim down a person who is overweight. To breathe correctly is normal . . . and correct breathing brings one to normal . . . and helps keep you there.

To be alive and thrill with the joy of living you must learn to breathe correctly! You must learn to breathe with every cell of your lungs. It is then and only then that you raise your rate of physical vibration to its highest level.

You can burn off fat by internal combustion. You can firm your flesh and keep it firm . . . normalize your figure into its naturally pleasing curves . . . by correct breathing habits, along with brisk walking, exercise and a natural diet.

NO ONE CAN BREATHE FOR YOU

You can build a new figure . . . a new YOU, inside and out . . . vibrant, healthy, tingling with the joy of life. But remember . . . you and YOU ALONE have this power. No one can breathe for you!

And this power is no good unless it is used . . . and used every day.

By daily Super-Brain Breathing you can build perfect blood circulation. You will no longer feel fatigued at the least physical effort. You will not feel dopey or drugged after eating.

Daily Super-Brain Breathing will bring a sparkle to your eyes . . . a glow to your flesh . . . and vim and vigor in your step. You will be mentally alert. Your reflexes will work perfectly. You will be fit . . . and you will feel fit . . . and have that sense of wellbeing that is a far greater treasure than any material possessions.

The most valuable of all elements . . . oxygen . . . is the most freely to be obtained. You have only to learn how to utilize it fully by Super-Brain Breathing.

By practicing Super-Brain Breathing you will develop long, slow breathing at all times. Remember that the person who takes fewer but deeper breaths per minute enjoys greater health . . . more endurance . . . more vitality and energy . . . and a longer, more youthful life.

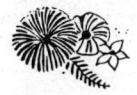

Chapter 6

Preparation For Super-Brain Breathing

Very few people can start the Super-Brain Breathing exercises at once. Most humans are the victims of bad habits of shallow breathing and incorrect posture. These habits must be overcome. Muscles must be strengthened, especially the diaphragm and the abdominal muscles. Unused air sacs must be opened.

Perhaps you have already experienced a *"stitch in the side"* when you have had to run to catch a bus or plane, or other unaccustomed exercise. Actually this is a good sign, if you will profit by it. It is good to exercise to the point of getting that "stitch". What it really means is that you have discovered a large area of unused lung cells, which have remained closed most of your life . . . since childhood games . . . and are now opening to receive the fresh air you are pumping in through extra efforts to breathe deeply.

These unused cells are slightly stuck together and collapsed upon themselves. The sharp pain is due to the air forcing them apart. Continue to breathe deeply, even if you have caught the bus or plane or stopped your exercise . . . the distress will pass, your unused cells will become activated, and you will have made an important step forward toward deep breathing and health.

Now, if you experience that "stitch" during the preparatory exercises which I am going to give you, you will understand what it is and not be alarmed. Just keep on breathing!

POSTURE EXERCISE

The principal value of correct posture is that the chest be expanded so that the lungs can be filled with air. As I have explained, the lungs themselves are passive in breathing . . . they are a collection of millions of tiny balloons which inflate with air when suction is created by action of the diaphragm and its auxilliary muscles of the chest and abdomen. The lungs cannot do this by themselves.

Remember, the lungs are attached to the walls of the rib cage by the pleural membrane. If the sternum, or breastbone, is carried high and the bony rib cage expanded, the lungs are held up in position so they can be filled with air. The uplifted diaphragm, in turn, tends to draw into position the sagging or prolapsed organs of the abdomen.

Most occupations today, however . . . from assembly line to desk . . . have a tendency to pull us down from an erect position. Many people carry the chest like a collapsed accordion, with the breastbone flat and the chest deflated, which again puts your heart and breathing apparatus in a vise-like grip.

To counteract this tendency, a special exercise is needed. Stand with toes and heels together. Now raise the hands overhead, at the same time rising high on the toes. See how high you can lift the chest . . . drawing in the abdomen. Stretch . . . stretch . . . try to touch the ceiling.

Repeat this posture exercise ten times. Do not try to do any special breathing. Just breathe naturally, or what is natural for you at the time.

This exercise is designed to strengthen the muscles which control the erect posture of the body. Stretching is one of the greatest forms of health building. It is the universal exercise of the animal kingdom. (Wild animals are beautiful creatures of natural living.)

After sitting for some time, always do this stretching exercise.

EXERCISING THE STOMACH MUSCLES

Most people have allowed their stomach muscles to become flabby. A good time to start strengthening these abdominal muscles and getting them under control is first thing in the morning, when you are in bed.

Lying on your back . . . with nothing over you but a thin sheet . . . fix your eyes and attention upon your abdomen. Now start a movement of its muscles . . . any kind of movement possible at first. Try to bring the contents of the abdomen upwards . . . then force them downwards. Wiggle your insides . . . toss them in one direction, then another . . . then from side to side. When you discover you can control them in one direction, practice that set of muscles . . . then try to get the muscles to twist and turn another way.

The point to reach is that of controlling your abdominal muscles in the same way you do those of your legs and arms. Your stomach muscles must do your bidding, if you want to develop a useful diaphragm.

After you have obtained some control over your stomach muscles while lying on your back in bed, *begin doing the same movements while standing upright.* In this position you can accomplish much more.

Upright, with hands passively hanging by the side of the body, draw up the contents of the abdomen until it looks like a deep valley . . . as though everything inside of you were up in the chest cavity. Then push them down until you are laughingly and innocently ashamed of your

protruding belly. Draw up . . . push down . . . wiggle, wobble, twist . . . turn all your insides over and around (at least, that is the feeling you should have).

When you have this will power over the abdominal muscles and contents, you will find that you will establish normal bowel rhythm. Outgo will equal intake, as it should . . . for each meal, there will be a bowel movement within an hour after eating.

DIAPHRAGM EXERCISE

In exercising your abdominal muscles, you will also be exercising your diaphragm . . . especially in the upward and downward pushing movements.

Now you should also do a special exercise for your diaphragm. First, *locate your diaphragm* by placing one hand at your waistline . . . then, holding the other palm upward in front of your mouth, blow imaginery dust from the palm. Where you feel a strong muscular contraction when blowing, that is your diaphragm . . . the most important muscle in correct breathing.

Now walk around your room on your tiptoes . . . with your hands reaching high over your head. Raise your diaphragm as high as your strength will allow you to lift it. Press it against your lungs and force out every bit of carbon-dioxide-laden air.

Then push your diaphragm down and out against the walls of your waistline . . . feeling it stretch the muscles of your chest and abdomen ... and suck in the oxygen-bearing fresh air into your lungs . . . with your chest lifted high.

If you feel a little dizzy at the oxygen stimulation, stop for a moment, then continue. *Start with 5 times . . . gradually increasing to 10.*

When you do this exercise with ease and pleasure, you are ready to start your Super-Brain Breathing Program.

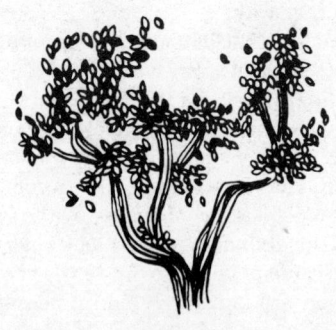

Chapter 7

What Is Super-Brain Breathing?

Super-Brain Breathing is a System of Breathing based upon simple, natural laws. The more oxygen you get into the body, the more carbon dioxide poison you will eliminate from the body. When oxygen replaces carbon dioxide there will be greater purity of the blood, cells and organs of the body.

It is a well known scientific fact that when all known modern methods of healing fail, the oxygen tent is used. Thousands upon thousands of lives have been saved in the oxygen tent.

Then let's reason this way . . . If a preponderance of oxygen can save the lives of humans who are on the brink of death . . . is it not logical that more oxygen can prolong our lives? . . . that it will free us from poisons that bring pain and distress to our physical bodies? . . . and, above all, give us a greater enjoyment in living?

Oxygen is the only stimulant upon which you can safely rely as a depression chaser and body builder.

Super-Brain Breathing has one purpose . . . and that is the forcing of more oxygen into all parts of the body.

Super-Brain Breathing Exercises should not be confused with physical exercises. While Super-Brain Breathing does produce physical and nervous strength, it has nothing to do with mere muscular development. However, it is almost impossible to have oxygen freely circulating in the body without beneficial effects showing in normal weight . . . hollows filling in . . . and improvement in the general tone and firmness of the flesh. Oxygen is absolutely the perfect normalizer.

The basic principle of Super-Brain Breathing is to fill the lungs to capacity with oxygen . . . hold the breath while leaning forward and dropping the head below the heart. This forces the oxygenized blood by force of gravity into the cavities of the head.

STIMULATION OF THE PITUITARY GLAND

The first and greatest benefit of Super-Brain Breathing Exercises is stimulation of the body's master gland, the pituitary. Located at the base of the brain, the pituitary gland is master of every human act and unconscious function occurring within the heart and abdominal cavity. Upon it depends the individual's height . . . length of bones . . . strength of muscles . . . calibre of mentality . . . pulse strength . . . term of existence.

Above all, the pituitary controls the functions of all the other glands of the body. It is *the master gland of life.* The more oxygenated blood you give the pituitary gland, the greater the output of all the valuable hormones of the body . . . the better the functioning of the glands, the more the body will rejuvenate itself.

That is why these seven exercises which I am going to give you are called Super-Brain Breathing Exercises. Although each is directed specifically toward a definite part of the body, all employ the same basic principle . . . and all stimulate the master pituitary gland.

EARLY MORNING IS THE BEST TIME FOR SUPER-BRAIN BREATHING EXERCISES

I recommend a 10-to-15-minute period early in the morning for your Super-Brain Breathing Exercises. After you have awakened your body with a few preliminary stretching exercises . . . sip a glass of water (preferably steam distilled) or fresh fruit or vegetable juice . . . then get ready to start your day with a peak supply of energy by Super-Brain Breathing.

The early morning hours are especially important for these exercises if you are a city-dweller . . . because the air is less polluted at this time of day than any other. Breathe that fresh air with its life-giving oxygen into your lungs before it becomes contaminated with poisonous fumes from the day's traffic and industrial operations. You will start your day with a glowing sense of wellbeing . . . and a store of energy to carry you through whatever work you have to do and problems you may meet.

Think of this period with pleasant anticipation . . . a time to build vitality, energy, strength and all the good things that come to a healthy body. What you put into this system of health building, you will get out of it. Go into it with all your heart and soul.

He who cannot find time for exercise, will have to find time for illness.

—Lord Derby

FRESH AIR AND WARMTH NECESSARY

Be sure that fresh air is circulating in your room . . . but don't try to do these exercises in too cold a room. I want you to get full benefit of this wonderful stimulation and to enjoy every minute of it.

If the room is cool when you get out of bed, put on something that is loose and warm. I use what is known in the athletic world as sweat shirt and sweat drawers . . . which you can find at any sporting goods store.

As you start doing your exercises, you will feel a wonderful glow coming over your entire body . . . and the more you breathe, the warmer you'll get. As soon as you feel warm enough . . . peel off the sweat clothes and get right down to your naked body. Give yourself an outside as well as inside air bath. Let the 96 million pores of your skin also breathe in the breath of life. Yes, indeed . . . you breathe through your skin, too! It's an important organ of respiration . . . your "third lung".

Those pores of your body will welcome a plunge into real fresh air. They are going to be wrapped up in clothes all day . . . and probably at night, too, unless you sleep in the raw as I do. A daily air bath does wonders for your skin . . . no creams or lotions can give you that "skin you love to touch" that fresh air does.

This will also greatly help your skin in its primary function as the thermostatic control of your body temperature. You will help condition it to meet hot and cold weather perfectly. It is a faithful thermostat when you give it a chance. But if you keep your body over-clothed and over-heated all the time, your skin becomes like a hot-house flower, unable to withstand drastic changes of temperature. When you allow your entire body to breathe freely in the nude, your thermostat will always work for you in either hot or cold.

BREATHE THROUGH THE MOUTH AND NOSE

Let me make it clear that in normal breathing, one should breathe through the nose. Nature has equipped this air passage with hair filters to strain out dust and soot . . . temperature regulating chambers (sinuses) to warm or cool the air before it enters the lungs . . . moist mucus to trap particles which pass through the hair filters and must be expelled through nose or mouth.

But Nature has also equipped the human body with a larger, secondary air entrance (the mouth) for use when a greater amount of oxygen is needed... as in strenuous exercise such as swimming, running.

Since the purpose of Super-Brain Breathing is to take into the lungs as much oxygen as possible, we use both the nose and the mouth to breathe it in. *Pucker the lips into a small opening,* so as to inhale slowly and strongly with a hissing sound.

PROCEED WITH CAUTION

Oxygen is a powerful stimulant. If your body has been on a starvation diet . . . as is the case with most humans . . . you can knock yourself out if you go about these Super-Brain Breathing Exercises too fast.

Proceed slowly. If you feel yourself getting dizzy . . . stop right then. After a few normal breaths you may feel like continuing . . . but it would probably be wise not to try to hold your breath to the full count of 10. Start with 5 if you wish . . . or with whatever number you are comfortable . . . and gradually increase to the full 10 count. After you start working on these exercises, you will be able to guage just how much oxygen stimulation you can take.

A note on counting: The "count" for holding your breath signifies the number of seconds. For correct timing, count "One thousand and one . . . one thousand and two . . ." and so on, so that one second should elapse with each count. And, of course, the counting should be done mentally — not vocally! Remember, you're holding your breath while you count — not expelling it.

MENTAL ATTITUDE IMPORTANT

I have already spoken about starting these exercises with pleasant anticipation . . . knowing that the result will be improvement in health and figure, and enjoyment in living a fuller, longer, more youthful life. Remember, your mind must be the boss of your body . . . and a positive mental attitude will bring you greater benefits sooner.

As you exhale, think to yourself, "I am expelling all poisons from my body . . . physical, mental and emotional. I am expelling sickness and fatigue, fear and hatred, envy and grief." Name whatever state of body, mind, emotions you want to get rid of, and feel that you are breathing it *out* of your system.

As you inhale, think to yourself, "I am breathing *in* health and strength . . . courage and self-confidence . . . love and peace of mind." Concentrate on the qualities you want to acquire, and feel that you are drawing these in with the fresh air and oxygen.

After you do this faithfully every day for several months, you will be amazed at how well it works. Your whole attitude toward life will improve. You will feel confident and happy . . . you will get along much better with your family and with other people, both friends and strangers. Petty annoyances will no longer bother you. Your worries and troubles will fall into proper perspective . . . you will be able to face your problems realistically and solve them with courage and ingenuity.

Let your mind and body work together in these Super-Brain Breathing Exercises . . . and living will become a glorious adventure!

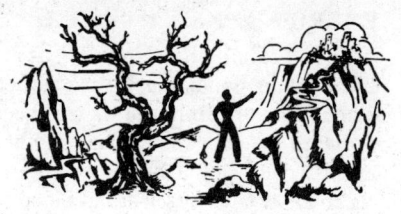

Chapter 8

Super-Brain Breathing Exercises

EXERCISE NO. 1 — CLEANSING BREATH

This is your basic Super-Brain Breathing Exercise.

Stand erect . . . feet about 18 inches apart . . . hands and arms relaxed at sides.

Raise the hands overhead. Now bend forward as far as possible . . . keeping the knees bent . . . at the same time exhaling through the mouth. Compress the chest and push upward with the diaphragm and abdominal muscles to expel every bit of carbon dioxide from your lungs.

Now slowly inhale through nose and mouth . . . pushing downward with your diaphragm and expanding your chest at front and sides to draw in the air to the full capacity of your lungs . . . as you return to the original standing position. As you do this, bring your arms upward in a half-circle to the overhead position.

(NOTE: All Super-Brain Breathing Exercises begin in this way.)

To complete the Cleansing Breath Exercise:

As your hands reach the overhead position . . . tighten your diaphragm and hold your breath for 4 or 5 seconds (mentally counting "One thousand and one . . . " etc.) while pulling your abdominal muscles back to "pin your stomach to your backbone."

Then exhale, bending forward as at the beginning . . . and inhale as you return to the starting position. Do this exercise 5 times.

33

EXERCISE No. 2 — THE SUPER-BRAIN BREATH

Start by exhaling and inhaling as at the beginning of Exercise No. 1.

When your hands reach the overhead position . . . hold your breath and bend forward from the waist, knees bent . . . dropping your head as far forward as you can. Continue to hold your breath to the count of 10 (mentally counting "One thousand and one . . ." etc.) . . . the purpose being to allow the oxygen-filled blood to suffuse the pituitary gland and reach and refresh every part of your brain, as well as cleanse the skull cavities (sinuses, ears, nose, mouth).

Still holding your breath, return to standing position . . . then bend forward, exhaling vigorously through the mouth. Slowly inhale as you return to starting position.

Do this exercise 5 times at the start . . . and gradually increase to 10 times.

NOTE: As previously mentioned, you may not be able to hold your breath for the full count at first. If you feel dizzy, exhale, return to standing position, drop arms to sides and relax for a minute or two before continuing the exercise. You will gradually build your oxygen tolerance to the full count.

EXERCISE No. 3 — SUPER-KIDNEY BREATH

Locate your kidneys on the lower back, just below the end of your rib cage near the waistline. Get the "feel" of them by placing your palms over this area, fingers and thumbs pointed downward . . . as this is the position you will take during the breath-holding part of this exercise.

Start by exhaling and inhaling as at the beginning of Exercise No. 1.

As your hands reach the overhead position . . . tighten your diaphragm and "pin your stomach to your backbone" with your abdominal muscles . . . while holding your breath. Now, still holding your breath, place palms over kidneys and bend forward . . . exerting a light pressure on the kidneys for a silent count of 10 ("One thousand and one . . ." etc.).

Still holding your breath, return to standing position . . . then bend forward, exhaling vigorously through the mouth. Slowly inhale as you return to starting position.

Do this exercise 5 times at the start . . . gradually increasing to 10. (Use same precaution in breath-holding count as given previously.)

EXERCISE No. 4 — BLOWING THE BOWEL

This exercise should be done in the bathroom on arising each morning . . . and several times within an hour after eating. If you will make this a habit, you will soon find that you will get a bowel movement within an hour after eating. This is as it should be . . . outgo should equal intake.

Start by exhaling and inhaling as at the beginning of Exercise No. 1.

Now, holding your breath, drop hands to sides in relaxed position ... and slowly go into a squatting position . . . then strain for a bowel movement for the silent count of several seconds.

Return to standing position and complete exercise by exhaling and inhaling as in previous exercises.

EXERCISE No. 5 — APEX OF LUNGS

This exercise is to get oxygen into the little used air sacs at the apex of the lungs, down near your waistline.

Exhale and inhale as at the start of Exercise No. 1 . . . but, instead of returning arms to overhead position, drop them relaxed at sides . . . and bring feet together, toes and heels touching.

Holding your breath, bend to the right and try to touch the floor with the fingers of your right hand . . . at the same time bringing the left hand up to touch under the left armpit. Hold position for a silent count of 10.

Return to starting position . . . exhale and inhale as before . . . then repeat breath-holding position on the left side, reaching toward the floor with the left hand, and touching the right hand under the right armpit . . . for a count of 10.

Return to starting position . . . exhale and inhale as before.

Do this exercise 5 to 10 times, alternating from side to side.

EXERCISE No. 6 — THE LIVER BREATH

Start by exhaling and inhaling as at the beginning of Exercise No. 1.

Now bring the feet together and clasp the fingers overhead, palms upward.

Keep legs stiff from the hips down . . . and holding the breath, bend slowly to the right side with as much stretch as possible . . . then to the left with a good stretch . . . alternating these bends to right and left 5 times each . . . while holding the breath.

Return to starting position with feet apart . . . exhale and inhale with the usual forward bend.

Do this exercise 5 times.

EXERCISE No. 7 — HEART STRENGTHENER

The purpose of this exercise is to expand the aorta, the main trunk of the arterial system which carries the blood from the heart after it has been oxygenized by Super-Brain Breathing. It stimulates the circulation of the blood in the heart, as well as throughout the rest of the body, helping to increase the power of the entire cardiovascular respiratory function. This exercise may give relief to those who suffer from angina pectoris, commonly called "choking in the chest", with feeling of suffocation and apprehension.

This exercise starts with the same exhaling and inhaling as in the beginning of Exercise No. 1 . . . except that the arms are held forward at shoulder height (not overhead).

When you return to the standing position, holding your breath . . . clasp your nose tightly with thumb and index finger so that no air can escape . . . and pretend you are blowing your nose. You should feel some air pressure in your ears.

Now, with knees bent, bend over from the waist . . . getting your head as near to the floor as possible . . . and continue to hold your breath for a silent count of 10.

Return to starting position and exhale and inhale in the usual Super-Brain Breathing manner.

Do this exercise 5 times.

FAITHFULNESS COUNTS

Every person who is interested in Super-Health . . . and who isn't? . . . should take time each morning to do these Super-Brain Breathing Excerises. Make it a daily habit. Make it as much a part of your life as dressing and brushing your teeth. The wonderful results you will obtain from faithfully following these exercises will repay your effort many times over in abundant health!

Take your present physical condition into consideration when you start on this program. Go slowly at first. A large part of your lungs has probably been dormant for a long time. It will take a while to open up these tissues.

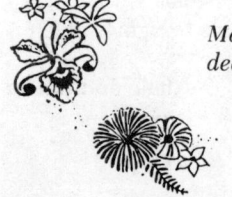

Man is composed of such elements as vital breath, deeds, thought, and the senses . . .

—*The Upanishads*

Chapter 9

Learn To Control Your Breathing

Remember, your lungs will hold six pints of air. If you keep your lungs filled to capacity you will feel better, have more energy, suffer less fatigue, sleep better, wake up faster, and be a happier person.

Learn to control your breathing so that you will take only 6 to 8 long, full breaths per minute. Long, full breaths fill up the lungs . . . and add healthy years to your life!

EVENING AND BEDTIME ROUTINES

At the end of the day's heavier activities, make it a habit to refresh yourself with diaphragm exercises and a few of the Super-Brain Breaths. Clear out from your body the ashes and cinders which have accumulated throughout the day. Make as much room as possible for air and good, natural food . . . then you will have a happy and relaxing evening.

Just before going to bed . . . after you have removed every stitch of clothing . . . stretch every inch of your body and exhale with vigor . . . and inhale with ease. Do not do any more. Get into bed and let the food of your evening meal be ground up, separated, and its valuable nutrients go to their places.

BREATHING TO RELIEVE PAIN

As civilized human beings, we tend to accumulate large amounts of latent poisons in our bodies. That means that Nature has concentrated toxic poisons in different parts of your body at periods during your life when these could not be disposed of through the regular avenues of elimination. These poisons are stored away in your veins, arteries, joints and organs. When these poisons press on the nerves, you feel pain. You may think this is something new . . . but, except in cases of direct injury, it is usually a "flare up" of old poisons.

Instead of merely taking a pill to ease the pain . . . a temporary expedient at best . . . why not get rid of the cause? Burn the poisons out of your body with oxygen! There is absolutely no better way of flushing the toxic poisons out of the body than by the powerful action of oxygen. Oxygen is the greatest purifier on earth!

For instance, you may have a pain in your right foot. That is quite natural, since by force of gravity poisons will many times seek the lowest level of the body.

Now let's get that poison out of that right foot. The technique is as follows: Lie flat on the floor . . . take a long, deep breath and hold it. While you are holding your breath, raise the left leg to the chest and with both hands press it against the chest . . . at the same time using the downward force of the diaphragm . . . and you will feel the oxygenated blood flowing down into the right foot.

This same technique may be applied to any part of the body. For a headache, for example: Take the full brain breath (exhaling and inhaling as at the start of Exercise No. 1) . . . holding the breath, lean as far forward as you can. This will allow a free flow of oxygenated blood to all the cavities of the head.

Aches and pains from fatigue are nearly always due to stagnant venous blood . . . filled with carbon dioxide . . . that is congested at various parts of the body. Swollen ankles, for instance, are generally due to an accumulation of venous blood. Exercise and deep breathing will help to activate the circulation and return this blood to the heart to be pumped to the lungs, where the carbon dioxide will be exchanged for purifying oxygen. If you have been sitting or standing for a long time and your ankles become swollen, lie flat on your back on the floor . . . raise your legs and stretch your feet toward the ceiling . . . and breathe deeply. You will feel the blood flowing from your feet and ankles toward your heart. If you are in a place where you cannot do this, breathe deeply and hold your breath . . . while you rise up on your toes, then down and up on your heels, alternately. The deep breathing and muscular action will stimulate circulation and relieve the venous blood congestion . . . and take the ache out of your feet!

RHYTHMIC BREATHING AND WALKING

Of all forms of exercise, brisk walking is the one that brings most of the body into action . . . it is the "king of exercise" . . . and when the rhythm of your breathing and the rhythm of your stride are in harmony, you feel like a king!

The Super-Brain Breathing Exercises in this book, when practiced faithfully, will give you such perfect control of your breathing that you can become a tireless walker. As the oxygen-filled blood courses through your body, your legs will carry you along buoyantly. Walk "tall" with head high, back and shoulders straight, chest out and tummy in . . . arms swinging easily from your shoulders . . . your legs moving smoothly as though they were attached to the middle of your torso.

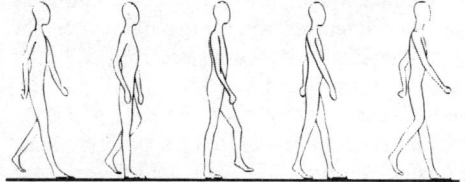

Walking posture. Always prepare a new base before leaving the old.

Enjoy your walk. Set your own pace, with a free spirit and a light heart. Watch with interest the things and people you pass . . . or let your walking be an accompaniment to your ideas and thoughts. As you breathe and walk rhythmically you lose awareness of your body, and you become as near poet and philosopher as you will ever be. You can truly "walk your worries away". As the blood courses through your arteries and veins cleansing and nourishing your entire body, you are filled with a sense of wellbeing that cleanses your mind of its troubles and nourishes it with positive thoughts. **Often as I stride along on my daily hike, I say to myself, "Health . . . Strength . . . Youth . . . Vitality."**

You should walk at least one mile every day . . . preferably more. Don't give yourself excuses. Make your daily walk a fixed item all the year around in any kind of weather. Walking requires no special equipment, and it can be done any time during your waking hours.

Although preferable outdoors, indoor walking is far better than none at all . . . in your hallway, on your porch or wherever you can get the most fresh air. When traveling around the world on my lecture tours, for example, I often take a late evening walk through the corridors and up and down the stairs of my hotel.

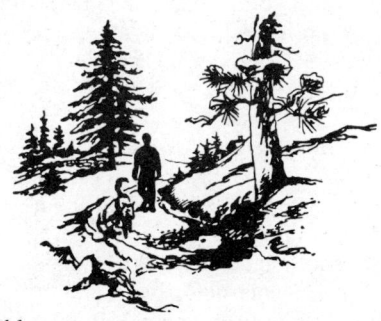

Life is like a game . . .
the chances are not in our power, but the playing is.
—*Terence*

CORRECT BREATHING
MAKES EXERCISE A PLEASURE

Whatever form of exercise you prefer . . . hiking, jogging, swimming, golfing, dancing, calisthentics, tennis, weight lifting, etc. . . . you will derive greater benefits because of the correct breathing habits which you will establish through this Super-Brain Breathing Program. What's more, you'll enjoy your exercise as never before!

My book, *"The Golden Keys To Internal Physical Fitness,"* will give you a basic Exercise Program, and so will the "Daily Dozen" Exercises in my *"Natural Method Of Physical Culture."* For Special Programs of Exercise, you might like to refer to such other Bragg Health Books as *"How To Keep The Heart Healthy And Fit"* . . . *"The Natural Way To Reduce"* . . . *"Building Strong Feet"* . . . *"The Fitness Program With Spine Motion"* . . . *"The Hollywood Beauty Plan"* . . . *"Preparing For Motherhood Nature's Way"* . . . all listed in the back of this book.

TRANQUILIZING EFFECT ON THE NERVES

The greatest tranquilizer for jangled nerves is deep, slow, diaphragmatic breathing. Today's tensions and pressures put additional strain on our nervous systems . . . and the condition is aggravated by poor posture habits and shallow breathing. Your Super-Brain Breathing Program will help you to correct both of these unhealthy habits . . . and will have a calming effect on your nerves.

During your workday, take at least a half-minute out of every hour to pause and s-t-r-e-t-c-h from the tips of your toes to the top of your head with deep, diaphragmatic breathing. The small amount of time invested in this will save you a great deal of time during the day, because you will be able to do your work faster and with greater efficiency. This is particularly important if you are a desk worker . . . but it is also helpful in any kind of work, even manual labor.

By oxygenating and relaxing your nerves, you will find that petty annoyances on the job, irritations with fellow workers or the boss, will disappear.

Whenever a big emotional upset occurs . . . as it inevitably does at times with all of us . . . go off by yourself and take long, full diaphragmatic breaths. See how few long, slow breaths you can take in a minute. You will find your nerves quieting down . . . logical thinking will replace emotionalism . . . and you will become master of the situation, able to solve your problem objectively.

For more details on this subject, you might like to consult my book on *"Building Powerful Nerve Force."*

RELIEF IN RESPIRATORY AILMENTS

Letters and case histories in my files give testimony of the blessed relief that Bragg Super-Brain Breathing has brought to literally thousands of sufferers from sinusitis, bronchitis, asthma and ephysema.

These "suffocating" diseases, which are characterized by inflamation of the mucous membranes with resultant obstruction of the air passages, are becoming more and more prevalent today as our air becomes more and more polluted. In fact, sinusitis . . . inflammation of the mucous membrane lining one or more of the sinus cavities in the head . . . is one the most common complaints brought to the doctor.

In bronchitis and asthma the mucous membrane of the bronchial tubes becomes inflamed. The human computer triggers the release of more mucus in an attempt to soothe and heal the irritation . . . but unless this mucus is decongested and expelled, it clogs these vital air passageways. In asthma, even the tiny bronchioles (the smallest branches of the bronchial tubes in the air sacs) become swollen. The victim feels as though he is suffocating — and in severe cases, he actually does.

Prolonged chronic bronchitis or asthma can progress into the dread emphysema, in which the air sacs become so distended with trapped air that this delicate tissue loses its vital elasticity. The air sacs themselves suffocate, one by one.

Super-Brain Breathing cannot restore the tissue that has been destroyed . . . but it can help to salvage and revitalize the rest of the lungs. The life-giving inflow of oxygen acts as a natural decongestant... gradually clearing the bronchioles and bronchial tubes . . . cleansing out carbon dioxide and other wastes from the air sacs and all the lung tissues . . . and revitalizing every cell with oxygen and nutrients.

Along with the super-brain breathing, it is absolutely essential that you eliminate all milk and milk products from your diet, as these are mucus-forming. This includes yogurt, cheeses of all kinds, ice cream, milk puddings, etc.

Many, many victims of these "suffocating" respiratory ailments have gained permanent relief by following a *complete health program* ... beginning with the elimination of milk and milk products and faithfully following the Bragg Super-Brain Breathing Program . . . gradually increasing the amount of brisk walking and other exercise . . . fasting for a 24-hour period every week . . . and following a strictly "live food" diet. In this connection, you will find helpful two of my other books, *"The Miracle Of Fasting"* and *"Toxicless Diet & Body Purification."*

Remember, as long as our lungs can extract enough oxygen from the air to cleanse the internal toxic poisons from our bodies, the human animal can survive and be healthy. Today, more than ever, correct breathing is a must!

Chapter 10

The Problem of Air Pollution

Practically every city of any size today faces the problem of polluted air. If you are a city dweller . . . as most people are . . . how are you to get the full benefit of oxygen under such conditions?

As previously recommended, do your Super-Brain Breathing Exercises early in the morning, when the air is least contaminated.

Also, especially if you live in a heavy smog area, install the best air filter you can find. That is what we used to do when we lived in Hollywood. Learn how to clean the filter and replace the pads, so it is always clean and washed . . . thus doing its job of cleaning and washing the air. Buy filter pads in long strips and cut them to fit as needed.

We recently sold our Hollywood home, because we did not want to be living in smog or any kind of polluted air even for short periods of time. If you are able to move away from pollution, do so! Your entire being benefits from fresh air!

CONSERVE OXYGEN WITH VITAMIN E

You should also fortify yourself internally with Vitamin E (natural d-alpha tocopherol), the body's "oxygen monitor". One of the vital functions of this "wonder vitamin" is to regulate the use of oxygen by the cells of the body . . . assuring that every bit of life-giving oxygen is properly utilized only for essential energy, with a reserve retained in the red corpuscles for use when extra effort is needed.

In this way Vitamin E increases the energy potential of every bit of oxygen you breathe by 50% to 250%, according to documented medical research.

I have certainly found this true in athletes who have trained under my instruction. Murray Rose, for example . . . the youngest Olympic triple gold medal winner in history, now the holder of six Olympic medals in distance swimming . . . takes a minimum of 200 I.U.'s of Vitamin E daily, increasing to 1500 I.U.'s during contests.

In fact, wheat germ, the prime source of Vitamin E, has become as much a part of the training of outstanding athletes as their daily workout.

Yet when I first advocated the necessity of Vitamin E supplements some 50 years ago, I was called a "faddist" and a "health nut". It is gratifying, of course, that today my premise has been substantiated by thorough scientific research, both laboratory and clinical, in the fields of biochemistry, nutrition and medicine . . . as well as by my own vigorous health as a great great-grandfather and that of many thousands of my health students all over the world, including famous stars in sports and motion pictures.

It is tragic, however, that it takes a half a century . . . and tens of thousands of needless deaths . . . as well as overall deterioration of health throughout the civilized world . . . for civilized man to realize that he robbed himself of the "staff of life" when he started making bread of refined white flour, stripped of wheat germ, the primary source of Vitamin E in the human diet.

It can be categorically stated that everyone who subsists on the standard "civilized" diet, devoid of whole grains but replete with refined white flour products, is suffering from Vitamin E deficiency. This means everyone of whatever age . . . infants, children, teenagers, adults.

This widespread Vitamin E deficiency has been documented as the prime factor in the disastrous increase in heart attacks and other cardiovascular problems. Two M.D. brothers, Drs. Evan and Wilfrid Shute, at the Shute Institute in London, Ontario, Canada, have conducted thorough clinical research over a period of more than 28 years ... treating more than 30,000 cardiovascular patients with massive doses of Vitamin E (alpha tocopherol) from natural sources . . . with amazing success. Their work has been confirmed, contributed to and extended by hundreds of physicians and biochemists throughout the world.

The primary functions of Vitamin E in the human body have been established as those regulating and maintaining the health of the entire cardiovascular system, vital to life. In connection with air pollution, the most important of these functions of Vitamin E is the conservations of oxygen within the body cells and bloodstream, as noted. This subject is currently being researched as an "antidote to smog" by Dr. Aloys L. Tappel, Biochemist Professor at the University of California at Davis. He also believes that this natural anti-oxidation property of Vitamin E can help reverse the aging process . . . and recommends that Vitamin E supplements be used from childhood on to help extend a healthy lifespan.

It has been suggested that this oxygen conservation quality of Vitamin E may also be effective in the relief or control of emphysema, the dread disease of lung deterioration which is becoming more prevalent as our air becomes more contaminated.

Vitamin E has proved to be amazingly effective in the treatment of burns of all degrees, and a Vitamin E salve is now available for home application to minor burns and sunburn.

ADD VITAMIN E TO YOUR DIET

Natural Vitamin E Supplements are available at Health Food Stores. If you are just starting on Vitamin E, doctors recommend that you begin with 100 I.U.'s daily, gradually increasing to 400 for women and 600 for men.

Wheat germ, of course, is the primary natural source of Vitamin E. Raw wheat germ may be purchased vacuum packed at your Health Food Store, also wheat germ oil. Both must be kept refrigerated immediately after opening! Wheat germ is highly perishable . . . that's why commercial millers refine it out of your flour . . . apparently being more interested in the shelf life of their product than in your life.

In the Bragg household, we sprinkle wheat germ over stewed or fresh fruit, and often use it in luncheon or dinner salads with raw, fresh vegetables. It has a pleasant, nutty taste. If you like the taste of wheat germ oil (some do, some don't), you will enjoy using it in your salad dressing. Mothers can even add wheat germ oil to the baby's milk. The two healthy children of that famous Hollywood couple, Clint and Maggie Eastwood, both like and thrive on wheat germ oil added to their goat's milk (1/2 to 1 teaspoon per cup).

If you're a bread eater, be sure to get only whole grain breads, which can be found at Health Foods Stores and at some special bakeries . . . or better still, if you have time, get whole grain, stone ground flour and bake your own. Patricia, my daughter, and I often do this, and it is really delicious!

Another rich food source of Vitamin E is cornmeal mush, made with 100% natural whole grain yellow cornmeal (not the degerminated variety found in most commercial markets). Here is Patricia's recipe:

Cornmeal Mush
1 cup 100% Natural Whole Grain Yellow Cornmeal
4 cups Water

Thicken meal with 1/2 cup of cold water. Heat balance of water to boiling, then slowly add the thickened cornmeal. Mix well. When evenly thickened, place in top of double boiler or in saucepan with heat turned very low, cook for 30 minutes (depending upon flavor desired).

Serve hot with honey, blackstrap molasses or (our favorite) 100% pure maple syrup. Or top with fresh fruit.

NOTE: If you are serving this to only 1 or 2 people, there will be some mush left over. Pour this into a flat pie tin, let it cool and put it into the refrigerator. For the next morning's breakfast, slice and dip in egg batter or roll in wheat germ. Brown in unsaturated oil (soya, safflower, corn, peanut, etc.) and serve hot with honey, blackstrap molasses or maple syrup.

FOODS RICH IN VITAMIN E

As you will see from the following table, compiled from lists in the authoritative *"Bridges Food & Beverage Analyses,"* a delicious variety of foods contain notable amounts of oxygen-saving Vitamin E.

Food	Quantity	Milligrams Vitamin E
Apples	1 medium	.74
Bananas	1 medium	.40
Barley	1/2 cup	3.2 to 5.2
Beans, Dry Navy	1/2 cup steamed	3.6
Beef Steak	1 average piece	.63
Beef Liver	1 average piece	1.4
Butter	6 tablespoons	2.4
Carrots	1 cup	.45
Celery, Green	1/2 cup	2.6
Chicken	3 slices	.25
Corn, Dried	1 cup	20.0
Cornmeal, Yellow	1/2 cup	1.7
Corn Oil	6 tablespoons	87.0
Eggs, Whole Fertile	2	2.0
Endive, Escarole	1/2 cup	2.0
Flour, Whole Grain	1 cup	54.0
Grapefruit	1/2	.52
Haddock	1 average piece	.39
Kale	1/2 cup	8.0
Lamb Chops	2 rib chops	.77
Lettuce	6 leaves	.5
Mackerel, canned	1/2 cup	165 to 250
Oatmeal, cooked	1/2 cup	2.0
Olive Oil	1/2 cup	3 to 8
Onions, raw	2 medium	.26
Oranges	1 small	.24
Parsley	1/2 cup	5.5
Peanuts	1/2 cup	26 to 36
Peanut Oil	6 tablespoons	22.0
Peas, Green	1 cup	2 to 6
Potatoes, White	1 medium	.06
Potatoes, Sweet	1 small	4.0
Rice, Brown	3/4 cup cooked	2.4
Rye	1/2 cup	2.2 to 3.5
Soybean Oil	6 tablespoons	140.0
Sunflower Seed	1/2 cup	31.0
Wheat Germ Oil (Crude)	6 tablespoons	150 to 420
Wheat Germ Oil (Medicinal)	6 tablespoons	320.0

EATING FOR OXYGEN

As shown in the foregoing table, the unsaturated oils ... preferably cold pressed ... are exceptionally rich in Vitamin E. Combine one of these (soya, corn, peanut, olive, etc.) with lemon or orange juice as a dressing for a combination raw vegetable salad ... and you will be eating both Vitamin E and oxygen.

Raw vegetables and fruits, in addition to their Vitamin E content, also contain large amounts of oxygen. Their juices have especially high oxygen content, being Nature's purest distilled water, H_2O.

All green leafy vegetables also supply you with the vital minerals, organic iron and copper, which are essential in the body's manufacture of hemoglobin. This is the substance in the red blood cells or corpuscles which enables them to absorb oxygen from the lungs and transport it to every part of the body.

Raw wheat germ, in addition to Vitamin E is also an important source of organic iron and copper. So are blackberries, raw spinach, fertile egg yolk, blackstrap molasses, sun-dried unsulphured apricots, raw nuts and seeds, dandelion greens, dates ... and the organs of animals, such as liver, heart, sweetbreads and brains.

About three-fifths of your daily diet should consist of raw fruits and vegetables. You can make many delicious combination salads and blender drinks for delightful and nutritious variety.

Although you also need cooked foods for a well balanced diet of natural nutrition, remember that cooking reduces and may eliminate the oxygen and vitamin content ... so never over-cook! Eat your meat rare ... and your vegetables lightly cooked in a minimum of water. Sun-dried fruits my be soaked overnight, or stewed over low heat.

You will find 1000 wonderful recipes for healthful, delicious and nutritious dishes in the *"Bragg New Generation Health Food Cook Book"* ... so you need never lack variety in your health menus.

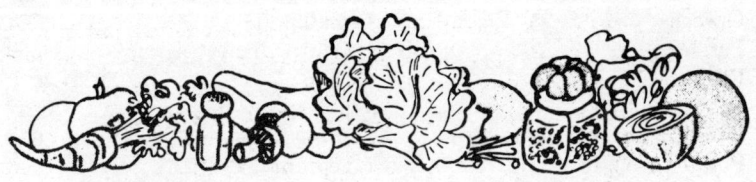

"Living under conditions of modern life, it is important to bear in mind that the preparation and refinement of food products either entirely eliminates or in part destroys the vital elements in the original material."
—*U.S. Dept. of Agriculture*

Chapter 11

Health Schedule of 12 Meals Per Week

Natural nutrition and correct breathing habits go hand in hand to lift you to high levels of vibration for happy, healthful living.

To attain and maintain the peak of Super Health, I believe in . . . and practice . . . an eating schedule of two meals per day, with a complete fast on distilled water alone for one 24-hour period each week.

As recommended earlier, I take a glass of distilled water or fruit juice before my morning Super-Brain Breathing Exercises. These are followed by about three hours of outdoor exercise . . . jogging, swimming, hiking, barbells, etc. Then I have a pick-up of fresh fruit and acidopholus milk or a nutritious blender drink, before getting to work on my writing.

My first real meal comes about midday. The reason for this is to give the stomach a thorough rest of 16 to 18 hours, allowing it time to completely empty itself, recuperate, and accumulate a goodly supply of digestive juices after the evening meal of the previous day.

LUNCHTIME IS SALAD TIME

Since most of us these days have a work schedule which does not permit a siesta after the midday meal (ideal if time allows for a short nap), we plan our main meal for the early evening and eat lightly at noon. You should never rush through any meal . . . relax and chew your food thoroughly, so the digestive process will get off to a good start and your food will be assimilated to give you the energy you need.

A full-meal salad of raw fruits or vegetables . . . with cheese, raw nuts or sunflower seeds for protein . . . makes an ideal luncheon. A favorite at the Bragg household is this recipe:

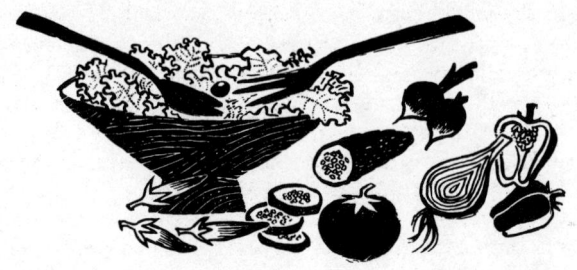

Bragg's Famous Vegetable Salad

1 stalk Celery, minced
¼ Green Pepper, minced
¼ Cucumber, minced
½ cup Cabbage, chopped

2 medium Tomatoes, chopped
3 Green Onions, chopped
1 large Avocado, mashed
A few sprigs Parsley, minced

Prepare vegetables as directed, and mix thoroughly. Serves 4.

In this combination you're "eating oxygen" along with vital vitamins and minerals and plenty of energy producing nourishment to carry you through a busy afternoon . . . and all in a flavorful combination to please your tastebuds.

(There are 54 different salad recipes and 23 for salad dressings in the "Bragg New Generation Health Food Cook Book".)

BALANCED VARIETY FOR DINNER

As previously recommended, relax at the end of your working day with a few Super-Brain Breaths and diaphragm exercises. Clean the day's poisons from your body so that you will get full benefit from a well balanced, nourishing and tasteful dinner! Your basic menu should include:

Salad . . . a smaller serving this time of fresh raw vegetables and/or fruits. Here are several suggestions: Cole slaw (grated cabbage) with diced green bell peppers and grated carrots . . . or grated carrots with fresh sliced apple or pineapple and raisins . . . or lettuce, tomato and cucumber salad. Make salad dressing of unsaturated oil and lemon or orange juice or natural cider vinegar. Sprinkle with wheat germ for taste and health.

Protein Dish . . . may be either animal or vegetable. Meat or eggs (fertile) should be eaten only 3 or 4 times per week, with vegetable proteins on other days . . . or you may adhere to a strictly vegetarian diet if you prefer. Meat should be lean lamb or beef, liver (broiled), chicken or turkey, fish (from non-mercury waters!). Eat your meat as rare as possible. Never use salt or condiments. Learn to prepare your meat dishes with fresh garlic, onions and herbs . . . and you will introduce yourself to a taste treat as well as health. Vegetable proteins include seeds (sunflower, pumpkin, sesame), avocado, soybeans, lima beans, lentils, raw nuts of all kinds (not salted).

Cooked Vegetables . . . should include one green and one yellow vegetable, lightly cooked. *No salt!* Cook in as little water as possible and only long enough for tasteful tenderness (5 to 15 minutes).

Dessert . . . should be fresh or stewed fruit, sweetened with honey, if desired.

For Super-Health, do not drink beverages with your meals . . . not even water! Let your digestive juices do their work undiluted.

Later in the evening, or at bedtime, have a cup of herb tea or a glass of fruit or vegetable juice, if you wish . . . and you may drink all the water, preferably steam distilled, that you wish between meals. But don't drink at mealtime!

DON'T POISON YOUR BODY
WITH FOODLESS FOODS AND HARMFUL DRINKS

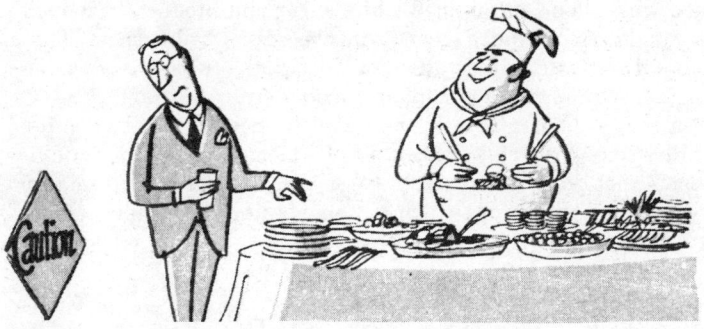

In our industrialized, urbanized civilization, we are paying a dear price for the convenience of mass distribution of foodstuffs. Not only has our flour been robbed of its vital wheat germ . . . but the great majority of commercialized foods have been rendered "foodless" . . . devitamized, demineralized, devitalized . . . in order to give them a longer "shelf life". You are risking your own life to eat these "foodless" foods that cannot nourish your body properly . . . and many of which **also contain preservative "additives" (such as nitrates and nitrites) whose cumulative effect has proved to be extremely harmful to the human body.**

Although the FDA (Federal Food & Drug Administration) has tried to protect the consumer by requiring the listing of most ingredients on processed, packaged and canned foods, few people bother to read the fine print . . . and if they do, seldom take the trouble to find out what the various preservatives or additives are. You don't have to be a chemist to find the answers . . . all you have to do is to use a modern dictionary.

For example, Webster's Collegiate Dictionary defines "nitrate" as "a salt or ester of nitric acid" . . . and defines "nitric acid" as "a corrosive liquid inorganic acid HNO_3 . ." Now, it doesn't require more than ordinary common sense to figure out what a steady diet of foods containing a concentrated form of a corrosive liquid inorganic acid is going to do to your body!

Sulphur (or sulfur) dioxide is another commercial preservative, commonly used on dried fruits . . . defined by Webster as "a heavy pungent gas SO_2, easily condensed to a colorless liquid and used esp. in making sulphuric acid . . ." Do I have to remind you that sulphuric acid eats away flesh?

Many fats such as margarines and even naturally unsaturated oils are ruined by being "hydrogenated" . . . a hardening process which keeps them from becoming rancid . . . but also makes them absolutely indigestible.

So read those labels and understand them. And strike from your market list all commercially refined and processed foods . . . such as refined white flour and refined white sugar and products made with these . . . processed "lunch meats" and cheeses . . . hydrogenated fats . . . foods with harmful preservatives or "additives" such as monosodium glutenate, sodium nitrate, sulphur dioxide, etc.

And . . . although these are not labeled "poison" . . . banish from your diet coffee, tea and alcohol, all of which do contain harmful ingredients that do become cumulative poisons in your body. Also avoid soft drinks and cola drinks which contain nothing but "empty calories" that can toxify your vital bloodstream.

DON'T USE SALT!

Salt was the first food preservative discovered by man . . . so many thousands of years ago that countless generations of "civilized" humans have believed salt to be a necessity of life. Primitive peoples know better . . . they don't use salt in their native diets . . . and they remain remarkably healthy, until they are discovered by civilized men and introduced to the poisons of civilization. Then their deterioration is rapid and tragic. I have seen this happen in the South Sea Islands, in Africa, in the Arctic.

The "salt of the earth" . . . inorganic sodium chloride . . . is poor food for plants . . . and poison for animals, including man. What about "salt licks"? Don't even wild animals "lick salt"? I investigated this quite thoroughly . . . and found that the natural so-called "salt licks" never contain sodium chloride . . . but are made up of organic minerals from decomposed plant life. And I regret to report that the commercial "salt licks" used by cattle raisers are for the purpose of making the beef cattle thirsty so they will drink a great deal of water, and therefore weigh more when they are sold. This is why meat so often "shrinks" excessively when you cook it.

All animals, including man, need minerals . . . but this need is for organic minerals, not inorganic. Only plants can digest inorganic minerals, which they take from the earth and by the process of photosynthesis convert into organic minerals to feed the animal kingdom. This is Nature's marvelous balance.

When our long-ago ancestors discovered that salt, or inorganic sodium chloride, would preserve meat from decay, they had no refrigeration or other means of storing food for long periods. And because they were extremely active physically, their bodies eliminated this indigestible inorganic mineral.

Civilized man today, however, is a sedentary creature. He does not eliminate the excessive amount of salt which he consumes . . . nor can his body assimilate it. So the body stashes it away . . . in crystals that harden the lining of the arteries and other blood vessels . . . in water solution that bloats the tissues and can ultimately cause congestive heart failure.

So . . . eliminate salt from your diet! If you think your food tastes "flat" without it . . . use powdered sea kelp, which has a tangy taste. Or take a lesson from famous French chefs . . . who use very little or no salt . . . but achieve their marvelous flavors by the skillful use of onions, garlic, mushrooms and herbs. Lemon juice is particularly good for seasoning meat and fish.

Salt actually deadens your tastebuds . . . without it, your tastebuds will awaken and you will enjoy the true, natural flavors of the food you eat. And even more important, you will feel better . . . and live longer!

FAST ONE DAY EACH WEEK

Oxygen, as I have stressed, is the greatest cleanser and purifier of the body. Give it a chance to do a thorough house-cleaning . . . to help the body rid itself of accumulated toxic poisons . . . by a 24-hour fast every week.

During this 24-hour period, drink plenty of steam distilled water . . . flavored with a little lemon juice and/or honey, if you wish . . . and nothing else! No food . . . no juices . . . no supplements. The only exception is a cup of herb tea . . . such as mint, alfalfa, anise seeds, etc. . . . if you feel the need of something warm inside.

Freed from the daily chore of digesting and assimilating food, your body will utilize its oxygen-given energy to cleanse itself thoroughly. Even after your first fast you will feel a renewed vitality . . . and as you make this a weekly habit, you will feel invigorated and rejuvenated.

I take my regular weekly fast from Monday evening to Tuesday evening. After my evening meal on Monday, I take nothing but steam distilled water until dinnertime on Tuesday. I have done this for more years than many people have lived . . . and I'm still going strong!

Several times each year I take a longer "super" fast, with nothing but distilled water for an entire week . . . and it works wonders in keeping me fit. If you would like to know more about the methods and benefits of scientific fasting, consult my book, *"The Miracle Of Fasting"*.

DRINK ONLY DISTILLED WATER

Not merely on your fast days . . . but every day of your life . . . let your drinking water be pure distilled water, preferably steam produced. You will be "drinking oxygen" with this pure H2O. In addition to fresh fruit and vegetable juices . . . which are naturally distilled . . . this is the only "safe" water to drink on this polluted planet of ours.

Even rain water . . . the ideal distilled water when it leaves the clouds . . . becomes contaminated as it passes through our polluted atmosphere.

Mineral water and ground water (from springs, wells, streams, etc.) contains inorganic minerals which are not assimilated by the body . . . and which can produce harmful deposits in the blood vessels, joints, kidneys and gall bladder.

Water from reservoirs . . . chemically treated to kill germs . . . contains harsh chemicals such as chlorine which are harmful to the body... plus inorganic minerals!

Water softeners only suspend these inorganic minerals, making the water more "sudsy"... but in no way "softening" the effect on your body.

For the health and longer life of you and your family use distilled water for drinking and cooking!

You will find the complete, documented report on the health hazards of ordinary water and the reasons for drinking only steam distilled water in my book, *"The Shocking Truth About Water!"*

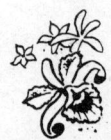

Chapter 12

A Strong Mind In A Strong Body

The great Greek civilization, which produced some of the greatest minds the world has ever known, lived by the motto, *"A strong mind in a strong body."* These ancient Greeks were noted not only for their amazing powers of endurance and healthy longevity, but also for their system of eating, deep breathing and exercising which produced physiques that have been models of art ever since.

The Greek system followed three main health principles:
1. Full and deep breathing.
2. Eating natural foods on the 2-meals-per-day schedule.
3. Systematized exercise for complete body development.

We can do the same and achieve the same results they did. We can become vital and totally fit . . . enjoying every minute of being alive.

The time to start is NOW . . . whatever your calendar years. Whether you are a teenager or a great-grandparent . . . or in between . . . it is never too early or too late to start on the Road to Super-Health!

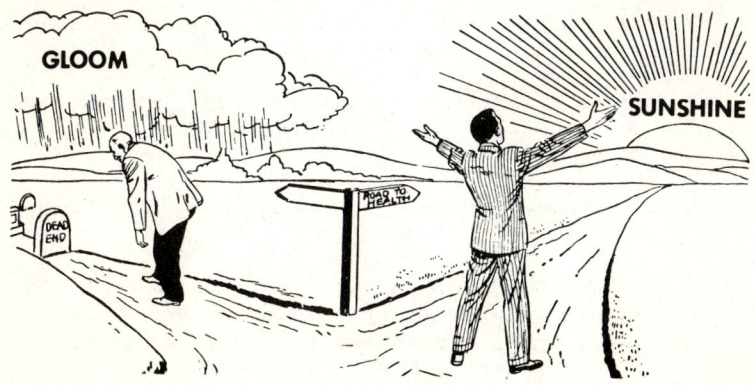

SUPER-OXYGEN FOR SUPER-LIVING

When the body is fed correctly with Live Foods and Super-Oxygen you thrill to the joy of living. Every day you bounce out of bed with that "glad to be alive" feeling . . . the feeling that there is a meaning to life.

When the body tingles from Super-Oxygen there are no depressed thoughts . . . no "down in the mouth" feeling . . . no envy, no hatreds, no jealousies . . . no blue Mondays, no frustrations . . . no fears, worries, anxieties . . . no morbid feelings.

With the stimulation of Super-Oxygen you are eager to meet life's problems . . . you meet them face to face and find solutions . . . you enjoy the effort of facing life's realities. You use the intelligence, reasoning power and common sense God gave you . . . to the fullest extent.

A person who knows how to breathe does not run away from life. He stands and faces it with courage and determination. The weakling who is a shallow breather takes the escape route . . . alcohol, drugs, self-pity . . . that can finally lead to the nightmare world of insanity.

Breath is life. Oxygen is your vital, invisible food. And Super-Oxygen gives you that tremendous stimulation which no other sustance can give.

THE ADVANTAGES OF SUPER-BRAIN BREATHING

Let us sum up the advantages of Super-Brain Breathing:

1. The most important of all physical acts is correct breathing. No one can be perfectly well and healthy who does not breathe deeply. Super-Brain Breathing Exercises help you to create the habit of correct breathing at all times.

2. When you breathe correctly you add millions of health-giving, oxygen-carrying red blood cells to your bloodstream.

3. When you fill the entire lungs with oxygen you cleanse your body of toxic poisons that could do you great damage.

4. Artificial stimulants are no longer craved when sufficient oxygen is taken into the system. Oxygen is absolutely the only stimulation that has no harmful after affects.

5. The more oxygen you get into your bloodstream, the more energy you have . . . the greater feeling of buoyancy and lightness.

6. Deep breathing is now a part of every cure. Today, the oxygen tent in the modern hospital wins many times when every other method of healing fails. Even broken bones heal more quickly when the blood is purified by daily breathing exercises.

Advantages of Super-Brain Breathing (continued):

7. Deep breathing is the great normalizer. Because oxygen is a food for the body . . . and causes perfect assimilation of other foods . . . the same deep breathing exercises will help both the underweight and the overweight to attain and maintain normal, healthy weight.

8. Super-Brain Breathing helps to make the weak strong, and the athlete a champion.

9. Many nervous diseases are due to oxygen starvation. Deep, diaphragmatic breathing tranquilizes jangled nerves . . . and also stimulates the brain to alertness and profound thought.

10. If everyone understood and practiced Super-Brain Breathing, there would be no need for eye, ear, nose and throat specialists. The oxygen filling these cavities destroys germs lodged there, and brings about a healthy circulation in these areas.

11. Many people suffer from poor circulation in various parts of the body . . . cold hands, cold feet, cold noses, cold ears . . . because they do not get sufficient oxygen to produce a steady circulation of the blood into these extremities. The more oxygen you get into your system, the better and more normal the circulation.

12. People who get sufficient oxygen have more tone to their muscles. The flesh looks more alive.

13. Oxygen is Nature's great beautifier . . . giving a radiant glow to the skin, lustrous sheen to the hair.

14. People who breathe in large amounts of oxygen are happy people. Deep breathing cleanses your body of psychological as well as physical poisons . . . and fills you with the joy of living and wellbeing.

15. Digestive ills are prevented or eliminated by internal massage of correct diaphragmatic action. Every time a Super-Brain Breath is taken the digestive tract is gently exercised.

16. Slow, deep breaths relieve the heart. Rapid, shallow breathing exhausts it by overwork and by lack of sufficient oxygen for the blood.

17. Probably the last thing one would expect to be influenced by correct breathing is straightening of the teeth. Yet most corrective work of the best dental colleges consists of deep diaphragmatic breathing. Correct breathing normalizes the cavities of the nose, mouth and throat, and exerts a gentle pressure upon the teeth.

18. Oxygen is the great food, stimulant and purifier which builds our resistance to infections . . . strengthens our weak points . . . is Nature's most vital aid in helping the body to heal itself . . . and to stay healthy. Better the ounce of prevention than the pound of cure! Breathe fully and live fully!

HEALTH IS YOUR BIRTHRIGHT — PROTECT & TREASURE IT!

This is a valuable book. Don't stop here . . . keep this book close to you and read and reread it until you get every health nugget it contains. Remember, you and you alone control your health, your life, and the way you look and feel!

Health comes from the inside out. It is true that you can be patched up after being stricken with disease, sickness and physical pain . . . but real 100% throbbing, vital health comes from your *good health habits*. That is the purpose of this book . . . to show you how to turn from the damaging habits which civilization has taught you.

Your health depends upon the way you conduct yourself each hour, each day, each week, each month, and each year. You are the sum total of your habits. It is true that your body can take a lot of punishment from bad habits. Sure, you can smoke, drink, eat dead, devitalized foods and apparently look and feel fine . . . yes, for a while . . . but you will have to balance your debts with Mother Nature someday.

And when something breaks . . . and you have heart trouble or one of the hundreds of other destroyers of health and life . . . it may be too late. It may mean a quick death . . . or years of living death.

I have no supernatural power to prevent or cure disease . . . that natural power is in your body. But modern science has discovered the way to live in health and happiness. I simply come to you only as a teacher, to tell you in as simple a way as possible what this modern science can do for you.

The rest is up to you. You have the method . . . it is now up to you to apply the intelligence that the Creator gave you. This is commonsense . . . and when something ceases to have commonsense, it ceases to be scientific. You have a treasure here, but only you can spend it. That treasure is the knowledge of healthful living.

* * * * * * * * *

Our sincere blessings to you dear friends, who make our lives so worthwhile and fulfilled by reading our teachings on natural living as our Creator laid down for us all to follow . . . Yes—he wants us all to follow the simple path of natural living and this is what we teach in our books and health crusades world-wide. Our prayers reach out to you for the best in health and happiness for you and your loved ones. This is the birthright He gives us all . . . but we must follow the laws He has laid down for us, so we can reap this precious health, physically, mentally and spiritually!

Paul C. Bragg   Patricia Bragg

"Teach me Thy way, O Lord;
and lead me in a plain path . . ."
Psalms 97:11

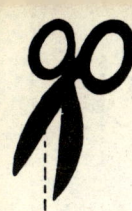

SEND FOR IMPORTANT FREE HEALTH BULLETINS

Patricia Bragg, from time to time sends News Bulletins on latest Health and Nutrition Discoveries. These are sent *free of charge!*

The Health Builder, the magazine devoted to Nutrition and Physical Fitness, is also sent *free* to those who are interested in gaining and maintaining superb health!

If you wish to receive these *free bulletins* and The Health Builder— please send your name and also names of any friends and relatives you wish.

HEALTH SCIENCE Box 7, Santa Barbara, California 93102 U.S.A.

Name

Address

City   State   Zip Code

Name

Address

City   State   Zip Code

Name

Address

City   State   Zip Code

Name

Address

City   State   Zip Code

PLEASE CUT ALONG DOTTED LINE

Please send Free Health Bulletins to these friends and relatives:

Name: _____

Address: _____

City: _____ State: _____ Zip Code: _____

Name: _____

Address: _____

City: _____ State: _____ Zip Code: _____

Name: _____

Address: _____

City: _____ State: _____ Zip Code: _____

Name: _____

Address: _____

City: _____ State: _____ Zip Code: _____

Name: _____

Address: _____

City: _____ State: _____ Zip Code: _____

Name: _____

Address: _____

City: _____ State: _____ Zip Code: _____

PLEASE CUT ALONG DOTTED LINE